# REFLEXOLOGY

### by Maybelle Segal, R.N., R.D., N.D., I.D.

Reflexology, or compression foot massage, is "a natural art of healing, a drugless way of stimulating the internal organs, thereby increasing the circulation and restoring bodily functions to normal." So says Maybelle Segal, a practitioner of this ancient art, one which was used as long ago in China as acupuncture. Revived in our country in 1913 by Dr. William Fitzgerald, reflexology has gained new adherents in recent times, many as a result of renewed interest in all natural preventive health measures.

But reflexology has also gained much attention because of the efforts Maybelle Segal has made to publicize this method. She has demonstrated compression foot massage on television and has won many converts to this healing art. And now she has written this basic book on the subject, intended for both the patient and the potential practitioner. It is an easy-to-read volume filled with helpful diagrams and photographs and written with a very personal touch.

Maybelle Segal is a woman devoted to her profession. She does not suggest that her patients not see their physicians. But she does think that today too many natural methods of healing are bypassed and too many drugs used.

Read about reflexology and see what you think. "Nature's way is God's way," says the author.

### About the Author

Maybelle Segal was born in Philadelphia, where she now resides. She is a graduate of the Hahnemann Hospital School of Nursing. She also has doctorates in reflexology, naturopathy, and iridology.

After many years in nursing, and after her husband's death, she felt that she could better serve mankind outside the hospital. In addition to her practice as a reflexologist, she is actively engaged in community health organizations.

Jacket Design and Illustr
by Gail Goldwater

D0964106

# REFLEXOLOGY

by Maybelle Segal, R.N., R.D., N.D., I.D.

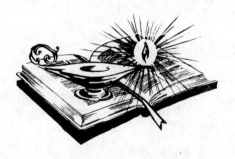

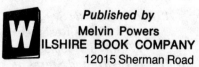

**Published by**
Melvin Powers
**WILSHIRE BOOK COMPANY**
12015 Sherman Road
No. Hollywood, California 91605
*Telephone: (213) 875-1711 / 983-1105*

*Printed by*

HAL LEIGHTON PRINTING COMPANY
P.O. Box 3952
North Hollywood, California 91605
Telephone: (213) 983-1105

Published from the original hardcover edition by arrangement with
Whitmore Publishing Company, Ardmore, Pennsylvania.

*To*
*God*
*The Great Physician*
*and to*
*All Mankind*

My sincere thanks to all of my family, friends, and patients, for each in his or her own way has contributed to the writing of this book.

# Contents

# Illustrations

*Figures*

## Plates

# Foreword

This book by Maybelle Segal removes the mystique from a procedure and profession that is receiving greater acclaim every day. It removes the veil surrounding compression foot massage, and bares for the nonprofessional—in easy to understand terms and testimony—convincing proof of a practice that deserves a much larger role in the nation's quest for good health.

The book reveals with unmistakable clarity the history, development, and increasing acceptance of reflexology. It carefully documents numerous benefits to be derived, and holds out new hope for people suffering with conditions that are being alleviated every day by this practice.

There is another dimension to this book that sets it apart from all other publications on the subject. This is the author's keen ability to look at the whole person and evaluate the negative impact of a poor diet. She explains the detrimental effect this can have upon a person, and how it can drastically reduce the positive benefits to be gained from foot massage.

As good health care increasingly becomes a luxury that fewer and fewer people can afford, it becomes incumbent upon Americans in all walks of life to explore this new reservoir of vitality nurtured by the proponents of reflexology. The author stresses this point repeatedly, and tells how a nonprofessional can, with conscientious effort and dedication, develop sufficient skill to practice on his or her own.

In the field of health care publications, Maybelle Segal brings to the public—through her book—more than literary talent.

Inbred in her text is a deep, underlying concern for human beings. To know her is a great privilege. To adopt her philosophy is a certain step to the pinnacle of good health. This book is a rare journey through that still unheralded maze called preventive health care.

Malcolm Poindexter,
TV News Correspondent and Commentator

# Introduction

Allow me to introduce you to the subject of reflexology. Known also as compression foot massage, reflexology is a natural art of healing. It is a natural and drugless way of stimulating the internal organs, thereby increasing the circulation and restoring bodily functions to normal.

Like acupuncture, reflexology has been used by the Chinese for 5,000 years. However, it was introduced to our medical profession in 1913, by Dr. William H. Fitzgerald, who graduated from the University of Vermont and served for many years on the staff of Boston City Hospital. At the time he brought reflexology to the attention of the medical field, he was active as the head of the nose and throat clinic at Saint Francis Hospital in Hartford, Connecticut. According to him, with proper application of pressure and massage to certain areas of the feet (relative to corresponding parts of the body), great stimulating, yet relaxing, effects can be noticed and enjoyed. Also, many bodily functions can be restored to normal.

If you are searching for help, trying to seek relief from nerve tension in your body, and trying to relax your body, reflexology might well be the answer to your problem. As you read and study this book, I hope you will be made to realize the great benefits which can be derived from this wonderful art of healing. Remember, this is Nature's way, and Nature's way is also God's way; and I believe that with God on your side, you cannot go wrong!

In the ensuing chapters, I shall try my best to explain, in

layman's language, the method of compression foot massage, parts of the body and corresponding areas on the feet, possible reactions (which, by the way, are natural reactions, far different from drug reactions), and some experiences and great challenges which I have had in reflexology. There will also be a chapter devoted to some of my patients, whose testimonials should help to convince you that there is much to be said for this wonderful healing art.

This book was written out of my deep concern for my fellowman, and much fasting and praying have accompanied the writing of it. I sincerely hope that my inspirations and feelings will be passed on to you.

I would like to think that in the near future reflexology will be more readily accepted by the medical profession (as it was when Dr. Fitzgerald first introduced it). After all, is it not true that all of us in the field of health should be working with one purpose in mind—that of restoring health to the ill? Would we not have greater accomplishments and success if we all worked together? If we just worked in harmony, I know we would better serve our nation!

After you have read this book, try to get some foot massages (to see what great results you, too, can obtain); then share it with your physician. Who knows? He may just read it and try it!

# Chapter 1

# Some of my Personal Feelings with Regard to Reflexology and the Medical Profession

I think of reflexology as a form of physical medicine, manipulation or use of hands being part of it. In physical medicine, methods are used to try to alleviate pain and discomfort. We, as reflexologists, do the same by trying to relax the patient and relieve nerve tension. It is my belief that reflexology should be part of the physical medicine department of every hospital.

It is most unfortunate that many a physician in the field of medicine will try to remove from competition anyone who helps people get well unless, of course, that individual is another licensed doctor of medicine. We reflexologists should not be a threat to any physician. Unless a physician is basically insecure, no one should pose a threat to him! In fact, if what I read is true, that the death rate of physicians from heart attacks is on the increase, these people should welcome our assistance. We are trying not to take away their patients, but merely to lighten the workload.

Yes, they tell us that about 80 percent of all the illnesses we suffer today are from tension and emotions. Then, if we, by compression foot massage, are able to relieve the tension and relax the individual, are we not being used also as instruments in the hands of God? And the wonderful thing about this natural way to restore health is that it is far superior to drugs, which years later leave their marks. I am aware that there are times when drugs must be used, but there are far too many times when the physician does not give Nature a chance.

3

The next time you have a headache, instead of taking aspirin (which *could* cause bleeding), try a foot massage and see if it doesn't work. Then on the next visit to your physician, tell him about your experience. He may give it some serious thought. After all, doctors can learn from their patients, too. Remember, this is how they got where they are today, by taking histories and doing physical examinations as far back as their medical student days. The theory they obtained in the classrooms, but the practice they received by actually caring for patients. An important part of their continuing education should be listening to patients with an open mind. No mind should be closed where patients are concerned. Life is too important to each and every one of us.

I pray that I may live to see the day when all of the professionals in the field of health will learn to work together, with one purpose in mind—*preventive health care*. Our first goal should be helping to heal the sick and prevent further illness. Instead, so many have as their first goal trying to make millions. This must detract from their concern for the patient.

If only all of the medical doctors, osteopathic doctors, naturopathic doctors, chiropractic doctors, doctors of reflexology, certified reflexologists, and others engaged in the art of healing would work together and in harmony, we would have a healthier nation because of it. If one in the healing arts cannot find the reason for the patient's problem, he should feel free to send the patient to another in the healing arts. This way, there would be a better chance of the patient's receiving the best care.

We live in a drug-oriented society, and because of this our nation is in a turmoil today. If more doctors would get patients away from drugs and lean more toward natural remedies, I think we would see a great change in our nation, a change for the better. Perhaps it is up to the patients to initiate this change. For too many years, doctors have been feared! It is time for you as a patient to speak up! Let your doctor know your feelings. If you are not pleased with your treatment or progress, let your doctor know. If you would feel more confident if another opinion were available, ask your doctor to call in a consultant. After all, if you do not express your feelings, your doctor will assume your progress is satisfactory to you. If more

4

patients talked to their doctors about natural remedies and their concern for preventive health care, I think more doctors would make a greater effort to practice preventive medicine.

You should also try organizing health groups in your church, synagogue, school, community, or even your home. Discuss openly your feelings concerning improvements which could be made in the field of health. There is so much material available for use. Take advantage of it. Push for better health programs! Write to your senators and congressmen, for I am sure they would help wherever possible. Isn't good health worth fighting for? Then don't delay; start today!

# Chapter 2

# Things to Remember about Reflexology

I learned something in basic nurses' training many years ago, but it stayed with me, and that is, that every patient who is physically ill is also mentally ill (meaning, of course, that the thinking capacity is impaired). If ever you have a physical ailment, you will realize, only too well, what this means. When you last had a cold, were you able to function properly? Did you not feel run-down, low, dragged-out, and as if you had cobwebs in your head? This was Nature's way of getting rid of poisons in your body, and giving it a good "housecleaning." After your cold was gone, did you not feel like a new person? It is extremely important to remember that the body works as a unit. When one part of the body is affected, the entire body suffers because of it. Reflexology works to relax the entire body and restore its functions to normal.

One may complain of a headache, constipation, and various other things, and when you start giving a foot massage to that person, you may be amazed to find the reflex to the liver to be very tender (which may mean it is sluggish). A sluggish liver may cause a headache and constipation. So, you see, at the same time you are massaging to restore normal function to the liver, you are also relieving the headache and the constipation.

Most times, after you have completed a foot massage, the patient will make the comment "I feel so relaxed, I could go right to sleep," or "I feel so great! I feel as if I'm walking on air." This is because you have increased the circulation, relieved the nerve tension, and relaxed the body completely. You do not have to go through life "uptight" because of the pressures of the world today. Just have a foot massage done, and see if it doesn't help you to better cope with your problems.

While the body is getting a "housecleaning," it is possible for reactions to occur. However, these are natural reactions, far different from drug reactions. These natural reactions will eventually subside, leaving no harmful effects, and your body will be better because of them. Let me mention just a few of these reactions, so that if you do encounter them, you will know there is no cause for alarm.

One patient came to me because she was having severe pain from sciatica, and no doctor could help her. She was told she had to "learn to live with it." This frightened her, because she did not know how she could endure this pain for the rest of her life. A friend suggested that she give reflexology a try. Because she was in such pain, she was willing to try anything. As I started to massage her feet, I found many areas to be tender. In fact, there were very few areas where I massaged that did not bring an "ouch" from her. All during the week following her treatment, she suffered from a cold (of course, this was Nature's way of ridding her body of toxins). The same thing happened after her next two treatments; but in spite of it, her sciatica greatly improved, and she was willing to put up with the discomforts of the cold. After her fourth treatment, she noted a remarkable change in her entire body. She said she felt as though she had been "made over." She now has treatments only occasionally.

I had another patient who came to the office because she was suffering from arthritis. She was also told by her doctor that she had to "learn to live with it." Of course, her doctor gave her medication to try to ease the pain; but when the drug wore off, she had the pain back again. I promised I would do my best to help give her some relief. But what I really do is help Nature along, so that she will have an easier time healing the body. After all, Nature *is* the one who does the healing! As I did the foot massage, I had to be ever so careful, because of her intense pain; but when the massage was completed, the patient really felt improved, and her pain was eased considerably. However, for three days following her treatment, she felt as though she

7

had been doing exercises for hours, her body ached so. She told me it was worth it, though, for as the body aches disappeared, so did her arthritic pains.

Some patients may perspire freely when getting a foot massage, while others may get slightly lightheaded. Of course, these reactions are caused because the body cannot accept the rapidity with which Nature gets rid of the toxins, and it reacts to this. If these reactions should occur while you are massaging, all you have to do is quickly massage the reflex area to the pituitary gland, which is the master gland. Effective results will be noted immediately. The reflex area to the pituitary is located approximately in the center of the big toe (see plate 1). It is the size of a pinhead, and usually with the correct amount of pressure you will be able to make contact with it.

While doing a foot massage, it is important to observe the facial expressions, the color, certain movements of the body, and the texture of the skin (whether it is cold and clammy or warm and dry). Quick observation will enable you to see if the patient is having a reaction. Stay calm. Do not become alarmed or panic. Remember, any reaction is a natural reaction, and it *will* subside, leaving no ill effects.

Here are some reactions noted by another reflexologist:

First, I would like to mention some reactions which occurred to me, after the first few massages I myself received. One was extreme tiredness and a sense of "lifelessness," which occurred after each of the first three massages; but following the third, I had a wonderful feeling of well-being. Another was that after the first massage, quite a bit of mucus was expectorated. Still another: a few days after the third one, there were several bowel movements, within a matter of a few hours—but not as diarrhea. Rather, they were well-formed, and afterwards I really felt well.

I have encountered other reactions. A friend of mine was having a problem with her left shoulder, and as I massaged the reflex area to the shoulder on her left foot, it was very, very tender. As I worked on it she mentioned that her left shoulder felt numb, and the numbness extended down her

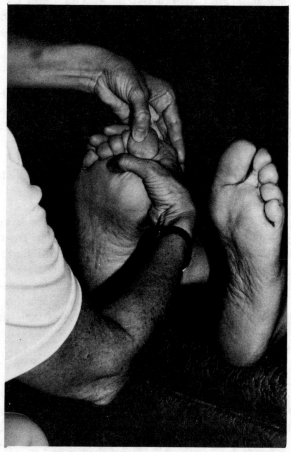

Plate 1. Reflex to the pituitary gland

arm. I continued to massage in that area and also did a few of the things often referred to by many reflexologists as "desserts"—which really help relax many being massaged. I also massaged the shoulder reflex area on her left hand. Within minutes the numb feeling was gone, and very shortly afterwards she remarked, "Oh, my shoulder is killing me." I continued her overall foot massage gently

9

and very soon after, completed it. As she stood on the floor, she exclaimed, "I don't believe it!" The severe pain she had suffered for over a month was gone and has never returned.

Occasionally someone has complained of cramps in the feet, which, after several "desserts," have disappeared.

At times, when working on someone suffering from sinus troubles, after "draining" the sinus reflex areas in the feet, the person has immediately found his (her) nose "running" freely (and stuffiness leaving).

The above experiences were related by Doris Young, a histology technician (ASCP).

There is no definite list of reactions which might occur, for each reflexologist has different experiences. It is good to keep in mind that each of us is an individual and should be treated as such. No two individuals are alike; so each will react in a different manner.

We reflexologists enjoy attending the seminars given frequently throughout the year. We not only learn from exchanging experiences, but we also learn from questions that are asked by new students. This way, we continue to stay abreast of new ideas and discoveries in the field of reflexology. One thing we all know is that so long as we live we should continue to learn. To stop learning is mental death.

It is wise for me to discuss at this time how often a massage should be done. The vital organs should have their reflex areas massaged once a week. In acute cases, they may be massaged every third day. They should not be massaged any more often, because these important organs must have a chance to recuperate from each housecleaning. Ridding the body of those poisons sometimes causes the body to become very fatigued, and three days' rest between massages will relieve this fatigue. Other parts of the body (the sinuses, the back, the head, the neck, the shoulder, etc.) may be massaged daily, even a few times a day if need be.

It is important to know that a complete foot massage should not be given for at least two days prior to a person's having a blood sugar test done. You see, when the reflex area to the liver

10

is massaged, the glycogen is released as sugar; this temporarily causes an elevation in the blood sugar. Also, massaging the reflex area to the pancreas will cause insulin to be released. And when the reflex area to the adrenal glands is massaged, the production of certain hormones alters the blood sugar level. The combination of all of these will temporarily render the blood sugar level inaccurate. In two days, however, the body itself will correct this. You can readily see that if a physician is regulating the dosage of medication according to the blood sugar results, the temporary "false" reading would pose a problem. We must always remember we are trying to work with the physician in every way possible.

Let me make you aware of the fact that drugs taken to alleviate pain may also render the tender spots on the feet much less tender. I usually ask patients who are taking such drugs not to take any before a treatment (unless, of course, it is specifically prescribed by the physician to be taken at regular intervals rather than only "whenever necessary"). But even if the patient has to take the drug and does not feel any tenderness while you are doing the foot massage, the massage will still be beneficial.

Another question which frequently arises is whether or not a conversation should take place while a foot massage is being done. There are some reflexologists who feel that a person receiving a foot massage is not completely relaxed if engaged in conversation while having a treatment. However, I find, once again, that each person must be treated as an individual. There are those who prefer simply to listen to soft music during the treatment; there are still others who have problems and would like to discuss them or get opinions on them while being treated. Of course, like all professional persons, we reflexologists keep these conversations between ourselves and the patients strictly confidential! This is extremely important, in that if it helps a person to talk about a problem, such conversation will also help to release some pent-up tension and relax the individual. I myself find that I am guided by the patient.

# Chapter 3

# Zone Identification

Dr. William Fitzgerald, the pioneer in reflexology, divided the body into ten zones vertically, five on the right side and five on the left side. Zone one begins in the thumb; travels up the hand, arm, shoulder, neck, and face, down the front *and* back of the body, extending down the leg to the foot, and terminates in the big toe. Zone two begins in the index finger and likewise travels through the body in the same direction and manner as zone one but terminates in the second toe. Zone three begins in the middle finger, travels through the body in the same manner as the other zones, and terminates in the third toe. Zone four begins in the ring finger, travels through the body in the same manner as the other zones, and terminates in the fourth toe. And zone five begins in the little finger and, like the others, travels through the body, then terminates in the little toe.

Organs or parts on the right side of the body have their reflex areas on the right foot and hand. Organs on the left side of the body have their reflex areas on the left foot and hand. Organs extending past the middle or center of the body will have reflex areas on both feet and hands. Where there are two like organs or parts (kidneys, ovaries, etc.), each has a reflex area on its corresponding foot and hand. The lower half of the body has its reflex areas on the lower half of the foot, and the upper half of the body has its reflex areas on the upper half of the foot. The waistline is located approximately halfway between the base of the toes and the lower part of the heel.

Do not become concerned if you have trouble trying to figure out where the corresponding areas are on the feet. If you get too "hung-up" on this, you will not be able to do justice to yourself or the person you are trying to help, whether he is a member of your family, a friend, or a patient. There is a simple way to help yourself learn the parts of the body. Purchase a simple anatomy book. Draw two feet the size of the book. Then take the drawings and place them alongside any illustrations in the book. The more you look at these, the more familiar you will become with the parts of the body and the areas on the feet. The combination of studying the charts and doing foot massages will help you fix the areas in your mind. Once you get to know them, you will not forget them. There is one point I would like to stress: regardless of where you find a tender area or spot, *work it out.* This will give the person you are massaging a tremendous amount of relief and relaxation!

You may purchase a few books on reflexology, and each one may have areas in a slightly different place. This may be because the author had his best results by massaging certain areas. This is why I must stress once again, no two people are alike; therefore, the reflex areas may vary slightly in each person. I have had patients who have told me they have unusual problems, such as a "dropped stomach," a "dropped transverse colon," a "dropped kidney," a prolapsed uterus, and even the heart on the *right* side. So you can see how the reflex areas to the various organs can vary. There is one sure thing: if you do a complete foot massage (covering every part of the foot, not missing so much as a fraction of an inch), you can be confident that good results will be obtained.

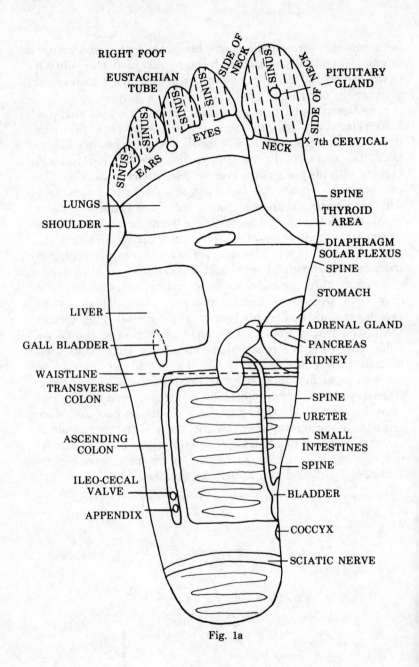

Fig. 1a

14

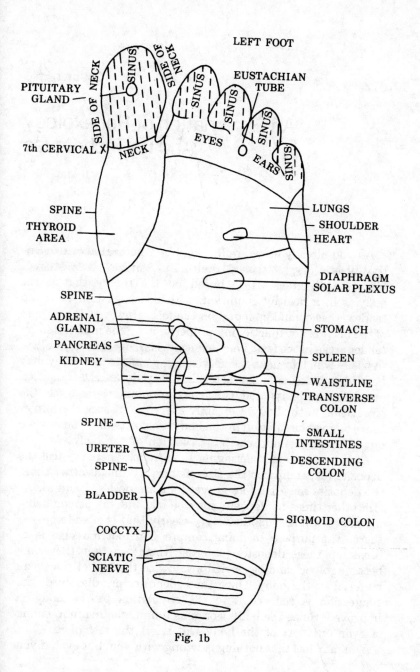

Fig. 1b

LEFT FOOT

PITUITARY GLAND

SIDE OF NECK

SINUS

SIDE OF NECK

SINUS

SINUS

EUSTACHIAN TUBE

SINUS

SINUS

7th CERVICAL X

NECK

EYES

EARS

SINUS

SPINE

THYROID AREA

LUNGS

SHOULDER

HEART

DIAPHRAGM SOLAR PLEXUS

SPINE

ADRENAL GLAND

PANCREAS

KIDNEY

STOMACH

SPLEEN

WAISTLINE

TRANSVERSE COLON

SPINE

URETER

SPINE

SMALL INTESTINES

DESCENDING COLON

BLADDER

COCCYX

SIGMOID COLON

SCIATIC NERVE

# Chapter 4

# An Explanation of Reflexology And Its Techniques

As you already know, reflexology is a natural and drugless way of stimulating the internal organs and increasing circulation to all areas. It is based on the theory that if the body is in a healthy condition, with no congestion in it, no tender areas should be found on the feet. However, if any part of the body is not functioning properly, it will be manifested by tender areas in the feet. This tenderness is caused by crystalline deposits which form at the nerve endings in the feet. They may be acid or alkaline in character, but they do denote congested areas in the body, and this congestion interferes with the circulation in the body. Certainly everyone realizes the importance of good circulation in the body. Deposits must be worked out in order to improve the circulation of the body.

At times a person massaging the feet may actually feel the deposits (depending on the size of them). While at other times the deposits may feel like gravel (but are no less painful). At still other times no deposits may be felt, but the person being massaged will let you know very clearly that the tenderness *is* there. The purpose in doing compression foot massage is to break up these deposits (or crush them) so that they may become solvent and be carried away with the rest of the waste material in the body. Once these deposits are dissolved, the congestion is relieved, and the circulation to the body is improved. Since the body works as a unit, the malfunctioning of even one part of the body will affect the rest of it.

You may feel that nothing is wrong with you, but even if you are only "uptight," your body is going to react to this. You may not realize it, but *Nature* will! Remember, Nature is the greatest educator in the world. Your body and mind can learn much from her, and the courses she teaches are free!

Let me now go into the techniques of compression foot massage. The first thing to do is to shorten your nails. They should be as short as possible, without causing soreness or tenderness to the tips of your thumbs or fingers. You can readily see why short nails are important; for massaging a tender area is painful enough, and long nails would just add to this discomfort. Also, massaging the tender areas many times brings the comment "You are digging your nails into me" (that is the feeling one gets often when the deposits are being crushed). Showing your short nails to the person will put his or her mind at ease. Also, be sure to wash your hands before and after each massage.

Now I shall describe one of the techniques, a caterpillar, or creeping motion. Although you will be using your thumbs a good deal of the time, you may find it easier to reach smaller areas with your fingers. This is fine, for it will give your thumbs a rest. Rest to them is extremely important, for overworking them or not using them properly may result in what is known as "trigger finger," a condition in which flexion (bending) or extension (straightening) is arrested temporarily but finally completed with a jerk. Take frequent periods of relaxation while you are learning the technique.

Ready? Take your right thumb, bend it, and place it on your left forearm. Now, using your thumb, push forward slightly, and at the same time straighten it. Now pull your thumb back slightly and at the same time bend it. Repeat this bending and straightening movement as you creep slowly up your arm. Using the side of the thumb many times makes for better results, for sometimes the pad of the thumb is too soft and may prevent you from giving the proper amount of pressure to make contact with the deposits (see plates 2 and 3).

It is most important to use pressure when massaging in order to make the right contact with the deposits, thereby helping them to dissolve. This does not mean that heavy pressure is used at all times. The amount of pressure varies, usually from

17

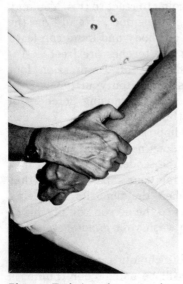 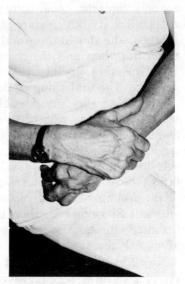

Plate 2. Technique for massaging    Plate 3. Technique for massaging

two to ten pounds. The amount you use will also depend upon various factors: the age of the patient, the severity of the tenderness in the area being massaged, the patient's tolerance to pain, and the general condition of the patient. You are probably thinking right now, "How do you know how much pressure you are exerting?" I found a very easy way to figure it. I practiced on my bathroom scale, using each finger individually, and going over it several times until I was sure I had the proper feel of it. Then to make doubly sure, I did it blindfolded, removing the blindfold with each finger and thumb to check my accuracy. The more I practiced, the easier it became, until I finally had it accomplished.

As you do more massaging every day, you will automatically become more familiar with the amount of pressure each person can tolerate. Just be sure you do not apply too much, for this may result in soreness and bruises to the area, and could prove to be very uncomfortable.

Bear in mind that all parts of the nervous system are bound

18

together by connective pathways; so massaging one area will also help to relax many other areas. Of course, one natural way of helping to remove the deposits is to walk barefoot every time the opportunity presents itself. This is exactly what was done for many centuries. Nature intended us to do just that; but we wear shoes thinking we are doing ourselves a favor, all the while encouraging deposits to form. Walking in your bare feet on the earth, sand, fields, stones, rocks, pebbles, etc., will allow these deposits to be crushed the natural way, with no help from anyone but Mother Nature. Of course, when going without shoes, beware of glass!

There are also devices which can be used for massaging, and some reflexologists say an eraser on the end of a pencil will suffice; however, in my experience, I have found no substitute for my fingers and thumbs. This is my personal opinion, but you may find that these devices will serve your purpose. Use whatever gives you the best results.

There is also a deep, rolling motion which I have found very beneficial, particularly when massaging the area for the sciatic nerve, the largest nerve in the body. You will find that your knuckles will play an important role in this rolling motion on many areas of the feet.

Let me make one strong statement. I am a firm believer in the fact that it does not matter what implements you use (if any, and if they are designed for this specific purpose) or what technique you use; what does matter is obtaining the desired results. If you find a method which gives you good results, then stay with it. After all, the end results are what really count. I say this because after you have been doing foot massages for a long while, you will pick up tricks and techniques of your own, and you will be amazed to see what great results you get.

In order to derive the greatest benefits from a foot massage, a person should be in a comfortable reclining chair with the feet elevated. He should have on no shoes, socks, or stockings. The reflexologist (or operator) should be seated in front of the person's feet. I have a massage chair which reclines and is quite comfortable for the patient, and at the same time, the feet are in a perfect position for massaging. There are times when you will probably have to do a massage with the person lying on a sofa, or on a bed. The important thing is to make sure both you and the person you are massaging are comfortable from the very beginning. An uncomfortable position prevents complete relaxation.

Many times corns and calluses prevent you from giving a good massage, for they prevent adequate contact with the deposits. I usually suggest that the patient arrange for a visit to her podiatrist before her next visit to my office, for this always makes for a better treatment.

In most of the plates and figures in this book, the feet will be pictured with the soles up. I mention this so you will realize that the right foot will be by the left hand of the operator, and the left foot will be by the right hand of the operator. Whenever possible, massage toward or in the direction of the heart.

# Chapter 5

# Reflexology and Diet

I feel that as beneficial as reflexology is, its benefits can be even more greatly realized if a proper diet and a good exercise program are used in conjunction with it. After all, we do say that if we help Nature along by trying to break up the deposits found in the feet, she will work with us. This is true, but if we break up deposits at one end to remove poisons and shove poisons in the other end, then we are defeating our purpose. Nautre *will* help us, but we must do our part. We are given much to work with; so let's make proper use of it. Remember, the body is the temple housing the soul. Treat it with respect and care.

It is very difficult to change a habit, and eating habits are no exception. Many times, if you force a change on a person, that person will rebel. For this reason, I try to use psychology to help a patient "unlearn" poor eating habits and learn new ones. I have a lending library available to my patients.

While a foot massage is being done, the subject of diet usually arises, and it is then that I begin to introduce the "unlearning" procedure. We discuss proper diet, and then I offer to lend the patient a book in order that he may become more familiar with the value and importance of good nutrition. Believe me, many a patient has found a whole new way of life through this self-education. People thus learn greater respect for their bodies. In turn, they give them better care. When you stop to think of it, we are our own best physicians, for who knows better than we how we really feel?

As for diet, I believe in the saying "We are what we eat." Most people eat with little thought of what takes place in the body during digestion. Let me mention, just briefly, some things which I hope will be of interest to you.

One extremely important thing to remember is that secretions of gastric juices, or fluids, is inhibited and digestion is delayed by anger, fear, worry, hatred, and many other emotional factors. Also, it is nice to know that active exercise increases the amount of blood in the skeletal muscles, thereby increasing the supply of blood to the stomach. For this reason, active exercise should not be taken too soon after a meal. The stomach should first be given a chance to help digestion along.

I try my best to use the correct food-combining diet. That means that I do not eat proteins and starches in the same meal. Starches require alkaline conditions for their digestion throughout the entire digestive tract; proteins require an acid treatment in their digestion in the stomach. Hence, if you combine starches and proteins in the same meal, the acid interferes with the alkaline and neither food is able to be digested. As a result, with starches, fermentation takes place and with protein, putrefaction (decomposition) takes place. Then come the dreaded symptoms of ptomaine poisoning, all too familiar to many of us.

I try my best to stay as close to natural foods as possible. I use fresh fruits and vegetables, unprocessed foods, and do not eat sugar or white flour. I do not drink fluids with my meals, since drinking with meals tends to dilute the gastric juices which are so important in the digestion of foods. If I drink water, I drink it at least fifteen minutes before my meal or between meals. I also drink herb teas frequently throughout the day. I take vitamin and mineral supplements, since in our polluted nation I consider them a necessity. Even fresh foods (organically grown) can be affected by the pollutants in our soil. Remember, airplanes give off vapor and gases which eventually wend their way into the ground.

In 1967 I found out I was a diabetic, and my physician started me on medication to lower my blood sugar (I took it reluctantly). It was discontinued after I suffered a bad reaction from it. I then consulted Dr. Evan Shute, who, along with his brother, Wilfrid Shute, runs the Shute Institute in Ontario, Canada. They have spent many, many years of research with Vitamin E (alpha tocopherol), and it has helped thousands of patients. Dr. Shute recommended that I start taking it. I did, and my diabetes has been under control.

There are many physicians who feel that vitamin and mineral supplements are not necessary. However, I know that I feel better when I take them. The minimum daily requirement suggested by the government does not appear to be sufficient for me. For this reason I have tried to find my own needs. I feel that, as I stated before, no two bodies are alike; therefore, we each should be treated individually. Too many times this individuality is ignored.

It is important for you to know that sugar and white flour are two culprits in the diets of many American people today. Sugar robs the body of calcium, and this loss of calcium can be the beginning of many ailments, arthritis being one of them. The sugar we use for our bodies is best obtained from natural sources such as fruits and vegetables.

Omitting sugar, white flour, processed foods, and refined foods from our diets can do much to help prevent disease, but we must also remember that the body needs a good cleansing regularly. By going on a good cleansing diet for a few days each month, you will give your liver a chance to become detoxified and rid it of poisons which have accumulated in it. I call my cleansing diet the "mono" or "duo" diet. In this diet, I use one or two kinds of food only, for three days. The food is usually a fruit in season. Watermelon is one of my favorites, because it is a cleanser and a purifier. I cut it up in small pieces and eat them frequently throughout the day. The three days I am on the cleansing diet, I take an herbal enema daily, to insure a complete body cleansing. On the fourth day, I gradually work in my regular diet until I have returned to my normal eating habits.

You mothers-to-be should remember to give your unborn children a chance to be healthy at birth. It is your responsibility, because they depend on you for proper food and nourishment for nine months. A healthy mother should deliver a healthy baby. After delivery, continue your good diet along with a good diet for the baby. As soon as your pediatrician places your baby on juices and strained foods, get busy with the strainer. Stay away from commercially prepared baby foods; they are loaded with poisons. You should use fresh squeezed juice and strained foods as close to natural as possible. Use the food you prepare for yourself; just strain it well. It may take you a little longer to prepare it; but your reward will be a happy, healthy baby.

I imagine there are people reading this book right now who have access to ground for planting but are not making use of it. Get busy! Make your own vegetable garden. It is a lot of work, but it is fun. And the end results are worth it! Do not forget to plant some herbs to be used as seasoning. To me there is nothing tastier than a fresh garden salad.

When I think of gardens, I think of a poem I learned as a child:

God's Garden
by Dorothy Frances Gurney

The kiss of the sun for pardon,
The song of the birds for mirth;
One is nearer God's Heart in a garden
Than anywhere else on earth.

# Chapter 6

# Headaches

Headaches, a common complaint of many, may be caused by almost any disturbance of a bodily function. They may be caused by gastrointestinal disturbances, the inhalation of impure air, allergies, eyestrain, emotions, stress, and some organic diseases. If a patient comes to me complaining of frequent headaches, my first concern is whether or not he or she has been seen by his or her family physician. Certainly medical advice should be obtained when persistent headaches are not relieved.

My patients have already seen physicians and have been given one of the following as a cause for the headaches: sinusitis, nerves, tension, pressure, eyestrain, or even upset stomach. Also, most of these patients have been given tranquilizers, analgesics, or a combination of the two to alleviate the pain. This may relieve the headache temporarily, but it does not get to the cause of it. For this reason, people seek further help. We many times refer to our patients as "medical rejects," for if all medical help fails, they turn to us as a last resort. A great many times this last resort works!

If most of the headaches are caused by everyday stress and strain, and if we are able to relax the patient by the use of reflexology, the headaches will be relieved. Many tension headaches can be relieved by massaging the top of the big toes (see plate 4). Be sure to massage the sides of the toes, for this is the neck reflex (see plate 5), and tension there most certainly may cause headaches. Massaging the outside of the big toes

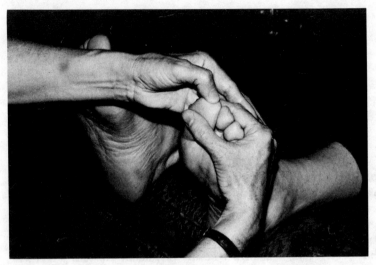

Plate 4. Reflex in the big toe to relieve tension

will relieve tension in the center of the neck, and massaging the inside of the big toe will relieve tension in the sides of the neck. This also reaches to the outer side of the head or brain. Massage to the base of the big toes will relieve tension in the back of the neck (see figure 2). Massaging the reflex to the seventh cervical vertebra (see plate 6) will do much to relieve that nerve tension.

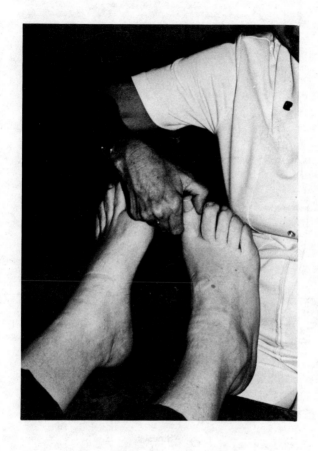

Plate 5. Reflex to the side of the neck

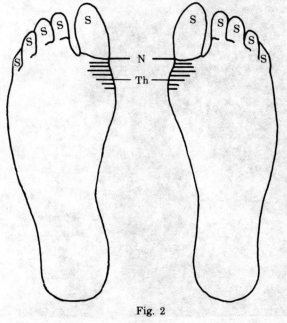

Fig. 2

S - Sinuses
N - Neck
Th - Throat

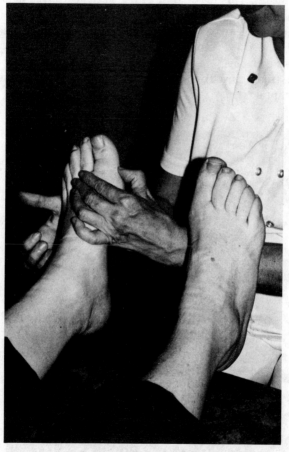

Plate 6. Reflex to the 7th cervical vertebra

Headaches caused by eyestrain may be relieved by massaging the base of the second and third toe. This is the reflex area to the eyes (see plate 7). Headaches associated with ear problems may be relieved by massaging the base of the fourth and fifth toes. This is the reflex area to the ears (see plate 8). If the headache is caused by a blocked eustachian tube (which leads from the ear to the throat), its reflex area will be found between the third and fourth toes at the base (see plate 9).

Sinus headaches may be relieved by massaging the balls of each toe (see figure 2). More about the sinuses is discussed in a later chapter.

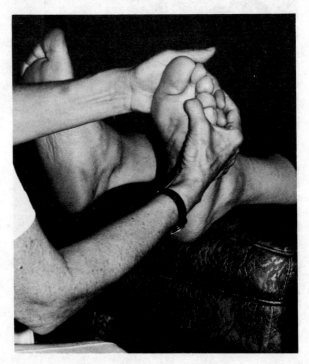

Plate 7. Reflex to the eyes

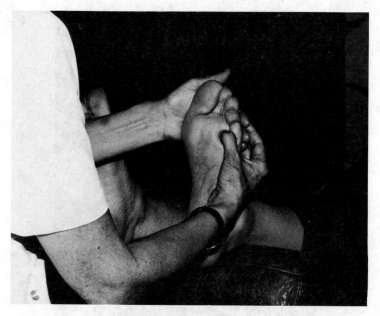

Plate 8. Reflex to the ears

Remember, as you are giving a complete foot massage, you are relaxing the entire body, and many times this will automatically get rid of the headache.

It is interesting to note that many people will get rid of a headache just by removing sugar from their diets. Yes, this is true. Headaches are a very common complaint among people suffering from low blood sugar. One patient stands out very vividly in my mind, for she was just a girl in her early twenties. Her supervisor (who knew me) sent her to me with the complaint of severe headaches. They were getting progressively worse, and she was becoming frantic. For four years she had been seeing a psychiatrist (a very reputable one, for I knew him well). He gave her tranquilizers to calm her and sleeping pills to help her get some rest, for he felt her problem was all emotional. This apparently was not the solution, for the medications did not seem to give her any relief. She came to me distraught,

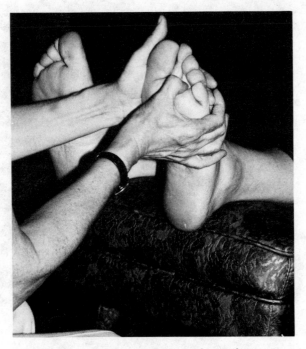

Plate 9. Reflex to the eustachian tube

depressed, and not knowing where to turn, for she felt that her condition was becoming worse. I first massaged her reflexes in her big toes to see if, at least, I could give her temporary relief from her severe headache. Her headache subsided within ten minutes, and I continued to do a complete foot massage. While working, I began asking her questions about her diet, for she seemed to have other symptoms associated with low blood sugar. She told me that she craved sweets, and, in fact, she felt as though she could not do without them. I offered her a book on low blood sugar, and she decided she would like to read it. My first suggestion was that, as of that moment, she try, as best as she could, to stay away from all foods containing sugar. Because she felt so miserable, she was willing to try anything that was suggested to her.

A few days later I received a telephone call from her and could tell by her voice that she was feeling much better. She said she felt as though she had been given a new lease on life. Not only were all of her symptoms gone, but she had not taken any medication since she had been given the massage and had started on a sugar-free diet. How wonderful to know that Nature can do so much for one so desperate!

Another type of headache which bears mentioning is a migraine. This type is extremely uncomfortable. Frequently it will occur on one side of the head and may be accompanied by gastrointestinal disturbances, disorders in vision, dizziness, sweating, chills, and sometimes even numbness and tingling in the extremities, particularly the hands, due to circulatory impairment. These headaches may last from a few hours to several days, and the symptoms may vary in severity. During a severe attack, a person is very sensitive to light and noise. Massage to both big toes may relieve the headache, but it is wise to do a complete foot massage in order to relieve the other symptoms associated with the migraine. If you have ever suffered with a migraine headache, then you are well aware of how the whole body is affected by it!

# Chapter 7

# Sinuses

The sinuses (cavities within a bone) are lined with mucous membrane, the same mucous membrane which lines the nose. When these membranes become inflamed, the condition is known as sinusitis. Sinusitis may be caused by many things: some are viruses, streptococci, staphylococci, pneumococci, dental abscesses, and a deviated septum. However, one of the most common causes of sinusitis is allergic reactions. These may include hay fever, rose fever, and many allergic maladies caused by airborne pollen.

The symptoms of sinusitis may include headache, nasal and postnasal discharge, toothache, pain behind the ears, and even pain in the neck. With acute sinusitis, a person may even suffer from chills, fever, and pain throughout the entire body. Symptoms usually vary with the sinuses affected.

I find many patients to be tender in the sinus reflexes, and yet they feel they have no problems with the sinuses. This is because they are under the impression that unless one has a postnasal discharge (drip), headache, or other specific symptoms associated with sinus problems, one is not suffering from irritated sinuses. As I question them, I find many of their complaints to be sinus related. As I massage the sinus reflexes, they find they can breathe more easily; then they realize their problems were caused by blocked sinuses. Within a matter of minutes after getting the sinus reflexes massaged, these patients reach for tissues to wipe their running noses.

There are several areas to massage on the feet, depending on

34

the associated symptons: the sides and the base of the big toe for the neck area and the ball of each toe for sinus blockage. Some reflexologists massage from right to left, beginning at the top of the toe and working the entire area to the base of the toe. However, I find that I get better drainage and results if I work lengthwise, from the top of the toe to the base, being sure the entire ball of each toe receives good massaging. Whatever gives you the better results is the method you should use. A good workout on the sides of the neck will also relieve congestion in the nasal passages.

Frontal headaches caused by irritated sinuses may be relieved by massaging the area just below the nail of the big toe (see figure 5). Amazingly, if you work the area from the nail to slightly below the base of the toe, you will also reach the reflex areas of the cheeks, teeth, and mouth. (A seven-year-old child came to my office one day for his weekly massage; I noticed he had a boil in the right corner of his mouth. It was quite inflamed, and the side of his face was very swollen. I concentrated for quite a while on this reflex on his foot, going back to it during the treatment. By the time he was ready to leave, the swelling was subsiding and the boil was becoming localized. I suggested that as soon as he arrived home he start to use hot compresses on it. In two days the boil was completely healed.)

The number of massages a person may require to relieve sinus problems will depend on many factors. The age and recuperative powers of the individual play an important part in this, as does the length of time the person has been "plagued" with the problem. Also, if the general health is good, the body should respond quickly to the foot massage. Most patients are relieved after the first or second treatment.

I have had some patients who have undergone surgery for the correction of sinus problems where the surgery was unsuccessful. With the help of a few foot massages, the problems were corrected.

To many, reflexology may seem too simple to work. But in my opinion, scientific proof or not, from firsthand experience, I know it works. I have seen too many wonderful results to question its value and worth.

# Chapter 8

# Asthma

Asthma, a most uncomfortable malady, is all too familiar to children and adults alike. Although there are a few types of asthma, the one most commonly known to the layman is bronchial asthma. It is usually due to a hypersensitivity to an allergen. Among the common allergens are inhalants (smoke, dust, pollen, and animal hair and foods (chocolate, strawberries, eggs, milk, fish, etc.). Infections of the respiratory tract (bronchitis and sinusitis) may also cause it. Emotional problems very frequently bring on attacks.

Some of the symptoms of asthma are shortness of breath, wheezing, a feeling of tightness in the chest, and a cough. The feeling of suffocation which frequently accompanies the attack causes the individual to panic; and this panic, in turn, only adds to the distress.

Two drugs of choice frequently used by the medical profession in the treatment of asthma are epinephrine (also known as adrenalin) and cortisone (and drugs related to it). Both of these are produced naturally by our own bodies. Therefore, if we can massage the feet and stimulate the body to produce its own adrenalin and cortisone, the results can be most rewarding. As I previously stated, Nature will heal the body for us if we but give her a little bit of assistance.

Every reflexologist has a different approach to the problem of asthma, but the end results are usually the same. I usually massage the pituitary gland first (since it is the master gland), then the adrenals (which manufacture the adrenalin and cortisone), then the thyroid gland (which helps to keep harmony with the other glands). Once the body begins to take over, within a short time the patient begins to get relief. However, while the massaging is being done, continuous reassurance must be given to the patient. I usually explain that Nature is working with us to help resolve the problem. It is important to assume a calm attitude in order to instill confidence. This calm is automatically transferred to the patient, and it becomes very noticeable.

My most rewarding experiences with asthmatics have been with children. If I have a child who comes into the office with an acute asthmatic attack, I work on the glands to get them started on their own. Then, after the child is quieted down, I let him listen to the mucus which is accumulated in the chest but loosened by the massage. I then explain the importance of coughing up this mucus in order to clear the lungs of this poison, making breathing easier. With a few minutes of "togetherness" (encouraging the child to cough), the child listens again to his chest (through the stethoscope), only to find the noise is gone. We call this a game, and it has helped many a child through an acute attack.

How thrilling it is to win the confidence of a child! Some of the parents tell me, "As soon as my child feels an attack coming, he asks if I will call you so he can have a foot massage done." The personal satisfaction I get, knowing I am doing my best to help people, cannot be measured in dollars and cents, for it is priceless.

# Chapter 9

# The Glands

A gland is a cell or a group of cells which takes certain material from the blood and makes substances with them. At the conclusion of this chapter you will find a chart which, I hope, will give you a clear understanding of the glands, their functions, their location in the body, and their reflex areas found on the feet.

The pituitary gland, also known as the master gland, has numerous functions. Because of the many hormones it secretes, it controls the growth of the skeleton, thyroid secretion, and regulates bodily processes such as reproduction and metabolic activities. It is a small, gray, rounded body, attached to the base of the brain. Its reflex area is located approximately in the center of the big toe (as you have already seen in plate 1). Sometimes a sensitive pituitary reflex will indicate hypertension, commonly known as high blood pressure. Massaging its reflex area can sometimes reduce this pressure and help normalize it.

The thyroid gland is located in the base of the neck, on both sides of the lower part of the larynx and upper part of the trachea, or windpipe. Its function is to control metabolic rate and normal growth and development; and it also stores iodine. A deficiency of the thyroid secretion results in a lowered metabolic rate in the body. Some problems caused by this are obesity, goiter, dry skin and hair, and sluggishness in all bodily functions. A person with an underactive thyroid is usually tired, not alert, has a slow pulse, and frequently suffers from low blood pressure. Since reflexology stimulates the internal secretions, it goes without saying that it tends to normalize the thyroid functions. Just as a deficiency in the thyroid results in the previously mentioned problems, an over-production of the secretion will tend to stimulate the basal metabolic rate, thus causing rapid pulse, weight loss, excitability, and sometimes psychic disturbances. Goiter, which is an enlargement of the thyroid gland may result from either an overactive or underactive thyroid, thyroiditis, inflammation from infections, and tumors. Whether you are dealing with any of these problems associated with the thyroid gland, reflexology tends to relax the individual and will help to normalize the functions of this gland. Its reflex area on the feet will be found below the big toe, in the first metatarsal area (see figure 3). Massage to this general area will also many times relieve a sore throat.

The parathyroid glands (four in number) are independent of the thyroid, but they are located on the back of and at the lower edge of the thyroid. They regulate the calcium-phosphorus metabolism. It is undersecretion of these glands which results in tetany (a nervous affliction). Some symptons associated with tetany are nervousness, muscle cramps, irritability, apprehension; sometimes even cataracts develop in these persons. The location of the parathyroids on the feet is in the same general area as the reflex area to the thyroid gland.

The pineal gland, attached to the roof of the brain, has no known function. However, since it secretes a hormone, it is still necessary to massage the reflex area in order that this secretion be produced readily. The location of its reflex area on the foot is at the upper aspect of the big toe, toward the second toe.

The adrenal glands, also known as the stress glands, are located adjacent to and covering the superior surface of the kidneys. The right adrenal is slightly smaller than the left one. Adrenalin is one of the hormones secreted by these glands. Remember, this is one hormone which does much to relieve one suffering from asthma. The steroid hormones (also used for asthmatics) are secreted by the adrenal cortex (the outer layers of the adrenals). Once again I say that reflexology is very beneficial in helping the body to produce these very important hormones.

39

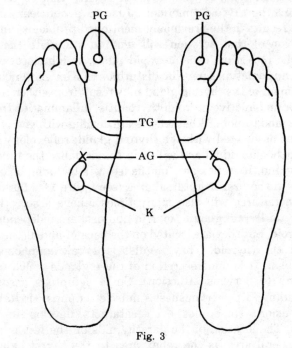

Fig. 3

PG - Pituitary Gland
TG - Thyroid Gland
AG - Adrenal Gland
K - Kidney

The adrenals also play a very vital role in enabling us to cope with our emergencies. They are responsible for giving us that "superhuman" strength which we receive at a time when the situation calls for it. Such strength can never be realized under normal conditions. Never underestimate the great work done by these glands. Their reflex area is located above the kidney area, between the first and second zones (see figure 3).

The ovary is the female reproductive gland responsible for the production of ova (eggs). It also produces two hormones, estrogen (a female hormone) and progesterone (responsible for the development of the placenta, or afterbirth, which provides nourishment for the fetus, or unborn child). The ovary is also responsible for the development of the mammary glands, or breast glands. There is one ovary on each side of the uterus, attached to the broad ligament, behind and below the uterine tubes. The reflex area to the ovary is located on the outside of each foot, midway between the edge of the heel and the ankle bone (see plate 10).

The testis is one of the two reproductive glands located in the scrotum (double pouch). It produces the male reproductive cells or sperm and also the male hormone testosterone. The reflex area to the testis is located in the same area as that of the ovary in the female.

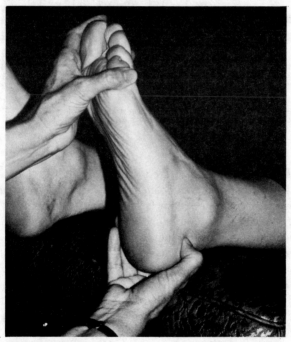

Plate 10. Reflex to the ovary (female) and testes (male)

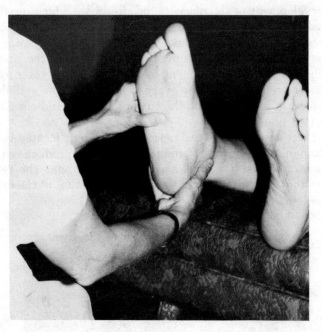

Plate 11. Reflex to the liver and gallbladder

The liver, the largest gland in the body, is located, or situated, on the right side beneath the diaphragm (the wall which separates the abdomen from the chest cavity). It is the first organ to receive blood from the intestines, where the blood has absorbed the final products of digestion. This vital organ removes glucose and stores it as glycogen. It is also a storage place for Vitamins A, B, D, and K. And is one of the main sources of body heat. Its reflex area on the foot is located below the pad in zones three, four, and five of the right foot. The gallbladder being on the undersurface of the liver, has its reflex area in the same general area as the liver (see plate 11).

The pancreas, located behind the stomach and in front of the first and second lumbar vertebrae (in a horizontal position), produces pancreatic juice, which is very important in the digestion of all foods. It also produces insulin, which is essential for the maintenance of proper blood sugar level. The reflex area to the pancreas is located on both feet (since it extends past the center of the body) and above the waistline (see plates 12 and 13). Since the pancreas is behind the stomach, it is hardly likely that you will be massaging its reflex without also including some of the stomach reflex.

Most diabetics and people with low blood sugar are very tender in the reflex area to the pancreas; however, bear in mind the fact that it is behind the stomach, the person being massaged may have stomach problems rather than problems with the pancreas. The complaints the person has will many times let you know which area is causing the problem.

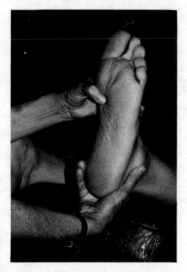

Plate 12. Reflex to the pancreas on the left foot

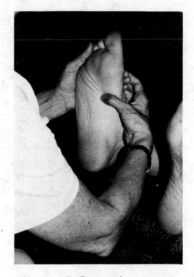

Plate 13. Reflex to the pancreas on the right foot

TABLE 1

The Glands: Their Function, Location, and Location of Reflex Area

| Gland | Function | Location in Body | Location on Foot |
|---|---|---|---|
| ADRENAL | Secretes hormones; helps one cope with emergencies. | One above the upper end of each kidney. | Above kidney area between the first and second zones. |
| LIVER | Storage place for glycogen, Vitamins A, B, D, K; source of body heat. | Under diaphragm, on right side, level with bottom of breast-bone. | Under pad of right foot, in zones three, four, and five. |
| OVARY | Produces ova, hormones. | One on each side of the uterus, behind and below tubes. | On outside area of each foot, midway between heel and anklebone. |
| PANCREAS | Secretes insulin; produces hormones for metabolism. | In front of first and second lumbar vertebrae, behind stomach. | Above waistline behind stomach area of zones one, two, and three (on both feet). |

44

| | | | |
|---|---|---|---|
| PARA-THYROIDS | Regulate blood calcium level. | Back surface of the thyroid (not part of it.) | Same general area as for thyroid (massage deeply). |
| PINEAL | Unknown. | Attached to roof of third ventricle (cavity) of brain (not part of it). | Upper aspect of each big toe, toward the second toe. |
| PITUITARY | Regulates body processes and metabolism. | Attached to base of brain. | Approximately in center of big toe. |
| TESTES | Secrete sperm and hormones. | Scrotum (double pouch). | On outside area of each foot, midway between heel and ankle-bone. |
| THYROID | Controls metabolic rate, growth, and development; stores iodine. | Base of neck, on both sides of lower part of larynx and upper part of trachea. | Zone one, in area of first metatarsal. |

# Chapter 10

# The Heart, Lungs, and Bronchial Tubes

The heart, a hollow, muscular organ, is located in the thorax, or chest cavity, between the lungs and above the diaphragm. It is the size of a closed fist and shaped like a blunt cone. Since the heart is the center of the circulatory system, it is extremely important to life. Without it, there is no life! As many of our problems are due to poor circulation, you can see how important it is to keep this organ in good working condition. Foot massages are certainly helpful in promoting good circulation. Since reflexology keeps the blood flowing freely, it does much to aid in preventing the formation of blood clots.

A thrombus, or blood clot, which obstructs a blood vessel or a cavity of the heart can be extremely dangerous. Many times, before a clot forms, the patient will develop inflammation of the vein, known as thrombophlebitis. Pain, redness, warmth in the area, and swelling may accompany this, and *under no circumstances* should this area be massaged! Loosening a clot could cause it to travel throughout the body, and lodge in the heart or lungs. *This could prove fatal.*

In the case of a blood clot or of thrombophlebitis (or of phlebitis, which is inflammation of a vein with no clot formation), the arm and hand of the side of the body on which the clot has formed can be massaged. The lower leg corresponds to the forearm, the upper leg to the upper arm, and the knee to the elbow. If the ankle is involved, then the wrist can be massaged. Massaging these corresponding areas can bring fantastic results. It is safe to massage the arm or its parts for

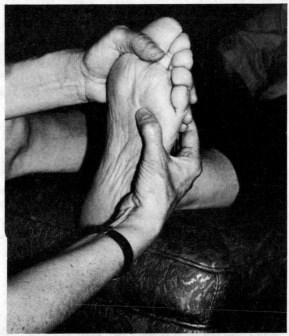

Plate 14. Reflex to the heart

the clot in the leg, for massaging the arm will not loosen the clot, but rather will help it to dissolve so that it can be absorbed in the bloodstream.

The reflex area to the heart is located on the left foot (the sole or pad), in the third and fourth zones (see plate 14). Be sure to take in a wide enough area when its reflex is massaged so as to better relax the heart muscle. One particular patient I have suffers from angina pectoris (pain about the heart radiating to the left shoulder, and sometimes even to the abdomen); and each time I give her the foot massage, she has the same experience. As I massage her heart reflex, she gets a feeling of fullness in her chest and sometimes a sharp pain down her left arm. After a few minutes, when the circulation begins to improve, the pain is gone and she is completely relaxed. She

47

truly feels that the foot massages are responsible for keeping her heart in good working order.

I have had patients who have experienced tenderness in the reflex to the heart, yet have never had heart problems. In all of these patients, I have found the blood pressure to be elevated. Once the massage is started and the patient begins to relax, the blood pressure is lowered, and the reflex area to the heart is no longer tender.

The lungs, also located in the thorax, are two cone-shaped spongelike organs of respiration. Their base rests on the diaphragm, and the top reaches to one inch above the collar-bone. The left lung has an indentation for the heart. Since the lungs take up a very large area in the chest, massaging the entire sole or pad of each foot will insure you complete coverage of them (see plate 15 for the general area). Working the entire pad will also loosen mucus and relieve congestion in the lungs. Relieving this congestion makes for a clear passageway for

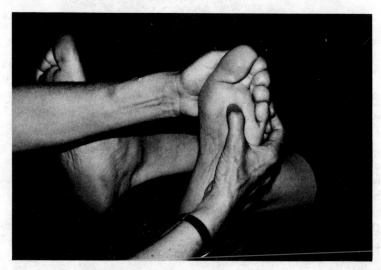

Plate 15. Reflex to the lungs

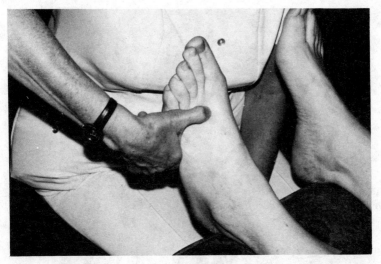

Plate 16. Reflex to the chest cavity, lungs breast (on upper surface of foot)

easier breathing. The upper surface of the foot (beginning at the base of the toes) also takes in the chest cavity, breast, and lung area (see plate 16).

The bronchi (two in number) are the primary divisions of the trachea, or windpipe. The right one is shorter than the left, and they penetrate the lungs (one for the left and one for the right). Then they divide into bronchioles and bronchial tubes. Massage to the reflex area of the bronchial tubes ("milking") can be a tremendous help in relieving a cough. Begin at the base of the sole of the foot (in the second and third zones) and pull (as you would pull the udders of a cow; the difference is that you are pulling upward on the foot). Place your thumb on the bottom of the foot and your index or middle finger (whichever is more comfortable for you) on the top of the foot. Then start pulling from the base of the sole of the foot to the base of the toes (see plate 17). I can remember one day when I was giving my niece a foot massage, she started coughing. I immediately started the milking motion, and she stopped coughing. She sat with her mouth wide-open, for she was in the middle of a cough and

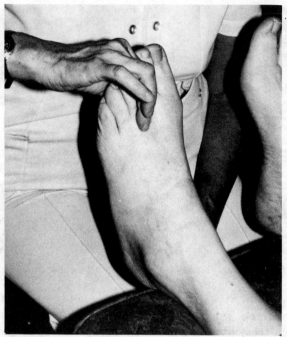

Plate 17. "Milking motion" used to open bronchial tubes

nothing happened! She had a look of amazement on her face, and from that day on she has reminded her parents, "Pull my feet if you hear me coughing during the night."

Before I close this chapter, I would like to mention something which many of my patients do in order to help rid the body of mucus. After having a foot massage, my patients go home and practice what is known as *postural drainage*. It is a position which one assumes in order to encourage drainage of secretions from the lungs and bronchial tubes. In this position, the head and chest are lower than the rest of the body. Lie with your body across the bed, the head and chest hanging over the side of the bed. A small stool is placed on the floor (put a pillow on the stool for more comfort) so that your crossed hands can rest on it. Tissues and a receptacle are placed beside it so as to

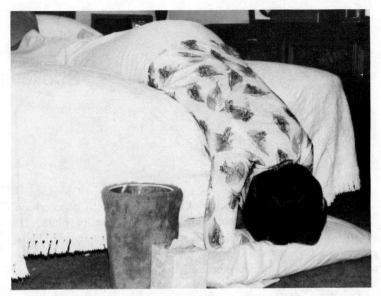

Plate 18. Position for "Postural Drainage"

properly dispose of the secretions or mucus (see plate 18). You then breathe deeply, turn from side to side, and cough. This does wonders for getting rid of secretions, and certainly improves breathing. One word of caution: This should be done for only ten or fifteen minutes at a time, and only three or four times a day. The position is very uncomfortable at first, but once you become accustomed to it, you will welcome the relief it gives you.

# Chapter 11

# Strokes

Stroke, also known as apoplexy, may be due to hemorrhage in the brain or spinal cord, or the formation of clots. Its symptoms may include headache, vomiting, convulsions, speech disturbances, difficulty in swallowing, loss of consciousness, and even coma. Remember, in cases of stroke, if there is hemorrhage in the right side of the brain, the left side of the body will be affected; and if there is hemorrhage to the left side of the brain, the right side of the body will be affected. But, when doing foot massages for a stroke, the right foot still takes care of the right side of the body, and the left foot still takes care of the left side of the body. This is important to remember, for paralysis of the right side of the body is aided if the right foot is massaged; and paralysis of the left side of the body is aided if the left foot is massaged.

Because of the severity of many strokes, foot massages may be given more often, but ever so lightly! Remember, all of the glands could be massaged more often, for they will help to regulate the bodily processes. Massaging the reflex area to the coccyx is extremely important, because of the possibility of the accumulation of blood in the spinal column (this would be due to hemorrhage). Do not forget the reflex area to the colon; this will help to regulate the bowels and rid the body of many toxins which have accumulated there.

Let me relate an experience I had with a very close friend of mine. As I went to his hospital room, his wife came to me and told me the physician had just been in, and said my friend had just suffered a massive stroke. He not only was in a deep coma, but was completely paralyzed. Just touching his skin, I knew he had a much elevated temperature, which made him extremely restless. I obtained permission from the nurse to give him sponge baths to help bring down his temperature (of course, this was my opportunity to give him a good foot massage!). I began massaging the reflex to his pituitary gland, for I knew this would help to normalize his bodily functions, and reduce his fever. Then I went to his adrenals and thyroid, because they produce important hormones. As I started to massage these reflexes, he began pulling his legs up toward his body. I was delighted to see this, for it proved to me that he was not completely paralyzed. He began mumbling, and I knew he was beginning to respond. I asked him if he was aware of my giving him a massage, and he mumbled yes and shook his head. I asked him if he wanted me to continue to do the massage, and again he shook his head yes. Within a half hour his fever was reduced, and I was able to aspirate (remove with a suction machine) much mucus which was in his chest, but loosened by the massage. His lungs were clear, and his breathing returned to normal. He quieted down and was very relaxed from his massage. For a few days, daily, I went to see him, and each day gave him another foot massage. In spite of my efforts, he did not recover; however, I did feel that at least I was able to make him a little more comfortable in his final days. If you do the best you can, then you should have no regrets.

Some stroke victims will respond to the point where they have little, if any, residual paralysis or speech impairment. This usually depends on the extent of damage and involvement. Remember, though, with extensive involvement in the body it may take longer for the body to fully respond. Do not give up, for many times your patience will be rewarded! These patients need encouragement; so be sure to give them the confidence they need to help weather the storm. It is truly a very thrilling experience to see stroke victims respond to foot massage.

# Chapter 12

# The Digestive System

The digestive tract is the digestive tube from the mouth to the rectum (see figure 4). It includes the mouth, pharynx, esophagus, stomach, small intestines, and large intestines. The accessory organs consist of the tongue, teeth, salivary glands, pancreas, and liver.

Most people do not stop to think that digestion begins in the mouth, with the proper chewing of food. You can readily understand, then, that any problems with the mouth, teeth, gums, or salivary glands will automatically get digestion off to a poor start; and the entire digestive system may be affected by this. Improperly fitted dentures, other dental problems, ulcers of the mouth, and diseases of these areas do not permit proper chewing. This may result in incomplete digestion and indigestion in many cases.

One of my patients had great problems with her dentures. Her gums were swollen, she had ulcers in her mouth, and she had difficulty in eating. This was further complicated by the fact that she was a diabetic, and eating was *extremely* vital to her well-being. When I started to massage her feet, I found many small deposits in the reflex area to her mouth. Because of her condition, I started light massage to this area, going back frequently during the course of the massage. The less painful it became, the more her body could tolerate and the deeper I could massage. After I was finished, she made another appointment for later in the week, for she felt that she needed it. The following morning she called to tell me that her gums were no

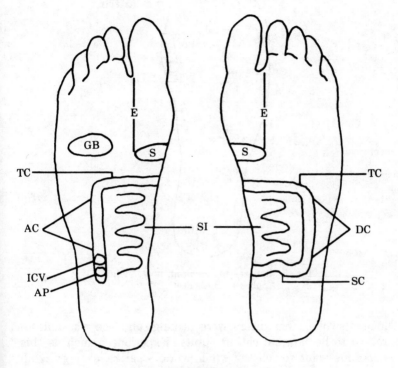

Fig. 4

E - Esophagus
S - Stomach
SI - Small Intestine
ICV - Ileo-Cecal Valve
AP - Appendix
AC - Ascending Colon
TC - Transverse Colon
DC - Descending Colon
SC - Sigmoid Colon
GB - Gall Bladder

55

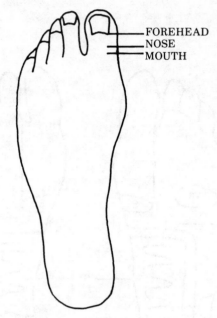

FOREHEAD
NOSE
MOUTH

Fig. 5 Reflexes for forehead, nose, mouth.
(Applies to Both Feet)

longer swollen, her ulcers were healing, and she was able to return to her normal eating habits. Experiences such as this make me want to tell the whole world what reflexology is all about.

As I explained before, the reflex area to the mouth and teeth will be found on the upper surface of the big toe. Begin working just below the toenail and continue all the way down to the base of the toe. At times it will be necessary to work even farther down the foot. In beginning below the toenail, if there is any infection from any of the sinuses in that area (remember, I said this could cause toothache), relieving any congestion there will bring great relief (see figure 5).

The esophagus is the canal extending from the pharynx to the stomach, and its primary function is, by wavelike movements, to pass the food on to the stomach. A person with a hiatal (or hiatus) hernia, which is a protrusion of the stomach upward, can have great discomfort in the region of the esophagus. Massage to its reflex area can bring much relief. Since the esophagus lies behind the trachea or windpipe, we would use the same milking motion which is used when massaging the reflex area to the bronchial tubes. You will marvel at how much relief this gives. In fact, I can remember when one of my patients "burped" for fifteen minutes after just this one area was massaged!

The stomach is situated below the esophagus, below the diaphragm, to the right of the spleen, and partly under the liver. Its functions are to hold the food while it undergoes certain mechanical and chemical changes which reduce it to a semiliquid form, to secrete gastric juices, and at frequent intervals to pass small amounts of partly digested food and digestive secretions into the intestines.

The shape and position of the stomach are modified by changes within itself and in the organs surrounding it. Since it extends past the center of the body, both feet are massaged in order to reach its entire area. Its reflex area is located below the diaphragm (which is just below the sole of the foot) and above the waistline on the inner aspect of both feet.

The small intestines, consisting of the duodenum, which is ten inches long; the jejunum, which is about eight feet long (this is also called the empty intestine because it is always found empty after death); and the ileum, which is twelve feet long (this is called the twisted intestine because of its numerous coils). The small intestines begin at the lower or pyloric end of the stomach and end at the ileocecal, or colic, valve. This valve prevents food material from reentering the small intestines.

The ileocecal valve plays a very important role in maladies in which a great amount of mucus accumulates in the body. Much of this mucus settles in the region of this valve and can cause much discomfort. Massage to its reflex area many times proves very painful because of accumulation of mucus and toxins in it. Relieving this congestion is of great benefit. The veriform appendix (a worm-shaped process projecting from the cecum) and the ileocecal valve are so close that massaging the reflex area to one will also help the other. This reflex area is located on the right foot, much below the waistline, toward the outer aspect of the foot, and above the heel.

It is in the small intestines, which receive bile and pancreatic fluid from the liver and pancreas, that the greatest amount of digestion and absorption takes place. Knowing this, one realizes the importance of keeping the small intestines in good working order. Their reflex area is located on both feet, beginning just below the waistline and extending above the heel. Taking in the areas of the first, second, third, and fourth zones will assure you that you have massaged the entire area to the small intestines.

The large intestines consist of the cecum (called the blind pouch), which is located below the entrance of the ileum at the ileocecal valve; the appendix; the colon, which is divided into the ascending, the transverse, the descending, and the sigmoid colons; the rectum; and the anus. In the large intestines the process of digestion is continued, the process of absorption is continued, and waste products are removed from the body. Massage to the colon reflex will help rid the body of poisons and unwanted bacteria. And often this massage will help to regulate the bowels.

In massaging the reflex area to the large intestines, I usually begin with the ileocecal valve, work up the ascending colon (to just below the waistline), over the transverse colon (which is continued on the left foot) and down the descending colon to the sigmoid colon. Since the sigmoid colon is in the shape of an S, as I reach the lower end of the descending colon, I work inward toward the inner aspect of the foot. This makes me feel a little more confident that I will make contact with the entire sigmoid colon. This reflex is important to many people who suffer from intestinal gas; for often they get a "gas pocket," or an accumulation of gas, in the sigmoid colon, which can be very distressing. Frequently, when I am massaging this area, a patient will say, "I feel gas moving in my abdomen." Of course, this is the stimulation of the gas which will either be expelled or dissolved.

Hemorrhoids (dilated blood vessels) can be relieved by massaging the reflex area to the rectum. It is located in the back of the leg, along the Achilles' tendon (this is the tendon so

58

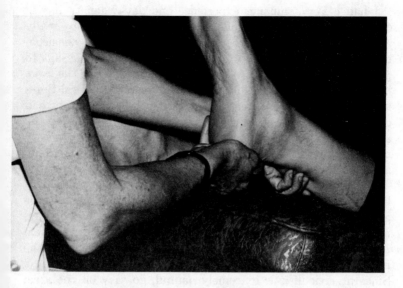

Plate 19. Reflex to the rectum, uterus, prostate gland, and sciatic nerve

frequently injured by ballplayers). Start at the back of the leg, at the same level as the anklebone, and work up a few inches (approximately four to six inches). Remember, though, if you find tenderness up still further, continue to work upward until you have been able to work the tender spots out (see plate 19). This reflex area is also massaged to relieve problems of the uterus, the prostate gland, and the sciatic nerve. Because this area is many times ever so tender, massage lightly, going back to it until it is relieved.

It is important to know that both diarrhea and constipation can be relieved by foot massage. Massage tends to increase the circulation, relax the muscles, and regulate the bowels. You see, you can have diarrhea and still suffer from constipation. The constipation will often cause a blockage, not allowing any fecal material to be eliminated. However, around the blocked fecal material liquid may seep, thus making one assume that one has diarrhea. Massage to the reflex area to the intestines will often correct this problem.

I had a very amusing experience one day when trying to convince a physician friend of mine that reflexology really works. Jokingly, he said to me, "If you can help my constipation, I'll be sold on it." I offered to give him a foot massage to prove that it would help. When I reached the area to the large intestines, I went over it, backward and forward, several times to get it working. For three days following the treatment he had diarrhea (Nature was once again getting rid of all of the accumulated toxins in his system). I began giving him weekly massages because he derived such great benefits from them, and it showed in his work.

Diverticulitis, a condition where there is inflammation of little sacs or pouches in the walls of the intestines, can also be greatly helped by foot massage. These pouches cause stagnation of feces, which, of course, causes congestion in the area. A foot massage will relieve this congestion by relaxing the muscles, and give these sacs or pouches a chance to empty. Since diverticulitis is extremely painful, go easy on the area.

The gallbladder is also another important part of the body which should be mentioned here. It is a pear-shaped sac on the undersurface of the liver; and although the liver secretes bile, the gallbladder stores it and discharges it into the duodenum as needed. Biliary colic can many times be relieved by simple foot massage. Also, gallstones may be crushed and dissolved by reflexology.

A neighbor of mine used to come to me for regular foot massages because of a back problem she was having. One day she came to my house and asked if I would give her a foot massage. She was having a problem, and the doctor felt she would need surgery. Her back was not the problem, but she did not tell me what the problem was, for she wanted to see if I could "pick it up on her feet." As I reached the gallbladder area, I could tell it was very tender. I turned to her and asked her if the doctor felt she should have her gallbladder removed. She had a look of amazement on her face; for although she had great faith in foot massage, her only real problem previously had been her back. This gallbladder problem was a new experience for her. I worked on it for quite a while until the tenderness was gone and she really felt relaxed. After the massage, her discomfort was gone. She was placed on a proper diet and has had no problems since. I am also very happy to say that she did not require surgery.

As I stated before, the reflex area to the gallbladder is just slightly below the reflex area to the liver on the right foot. Since it is on the undersurface of the liver, I will remind you once again that as you are working the liver area you are also helping the gallbladder (refresh your memory by checking plate 11 once again).

# Chapter 13

# The Urinary System

The urinary system is made up of two kidneys, two ureters, and the bladder (see figure 6). The kidneys are located at the back of the abdominal cavity, one on each side of the spinal column. Their function is to excrete waste matter in the body in the form of urine. The right kidney is a little lower than the left, because of the large space occupied by the liver.

It is the kidneys which help keep the body fluids normal in composition and volume by removing variable amounts of water and organic and inorganic substances from the bloodstream as it passes through them. They also remove foreign substances such as toxins. Accumulation of some of these substances can cause kidney stones, which are actually crystalline deposits (crystalline urinary salts). With a good foot massage, you will be able to relax the urinary tract, thus enabling a person to better pass a stone.

There are times when a kidney stone becomes lodged in the ureter (the tube carrying urine from the kidney to the bladder), and it is thus very difficult to pass. However, I have seen cases in which good results have been achieved through massaging the foot to help dissolve the stone. Oftentimes the patient has passed the stone and has had no further pain or complications.

The bladder, which acts as a reservoir for urine, can become easily inflamed. This condition is sometimes called cystitis. Cystitis occurs frequently in females because of improper care after urination. Although it is not usually dangerous, it can be very uncomfortable, carrying with it the symptoms of pain, pus, and frequency of urination. Little girls may also be bothered by this problem, and I can remember a pediatrician who taught us this in class in my student days. His statement was, "You will never forget the symptoms of cystitis if you will just remember the three P's" (meaning, of course, pain, pus, and plenty of urine!).

In massaging the reflex areas to the urinary system, I usually begin at the bladder area, go up the ureter area, and then to the kidney area. Then I retrace my steps, going from the kidney to the ureter, then down to the bladder. As I massage the kidney, I will also do the area of the adrenal gland, since it is adjacent to, and covers, the superior surface of the kidney. As I retrace my steps downward, I know that the kidney is stimulated to

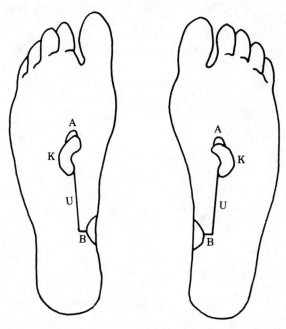

Fig. 6

B - Bladder
U - Ureter
K - Kidney
A - Adrenal Gland

send any excess urine down the ureter to the bladder, and when
the bladder is emptied, the system is cleansed and is ready to
begin its work again.

# Chapter 14

# Sciatica

The sciatic nerves (one on each side of the body) are the longest nerves in the body. They arise from the sacral plexus (which is a network of nerves in the area of the sacrum—the base of the vertebral column) and extend near the center of each buttock and the back of each thigh, to the region behind the knee. There each divides into two large branches which supply the leg and the foot.

Sciatica (also known as sciatic neuralgia) is inflammation of the sciatic nerve in which there is severe pain in the leg along the course of the nerve. It can be the result of trauma or of metabolic, toxic, or infectious disorders. This pain can also be referred to the sciatic nerve from other parts of the body. The pain may begin abruptly or gradually, and is usually a sharp, shooting pain beginning at the buttock and running down the back of the thigh. Movement of the leg may cause more intense pain, and it may be distributed along the entire leg or only in certain areas of it.

Sciatica may be accompanied by numbness and tingling, and the nerve may be extremely sensitive to the touch. The pain may be more intense at night and in damp weather. The number of foot massages needed to bring relief from that terrible pain will usually depend upon the severity and duration of the attack. The sooner a massage is given after the onset of the attack, the better the chances are that it will respond to the first treatment. I have never seen a patient who suffered from sciatica not respond to reflexology. In chapter 21 you will read

of a very well known TV personality in the Philadelphia area
who certainly attests to its great worth in this regard.

There are several areas which can be massaged to bring relief
from the pain from sciatica. One was previously mentioned in
chapter 12, that is the back of the leg. Another area is behind
the outside anklebone of each foot (see plate 20). Still another
area which can be massaged is found along the outside edge of
the foot. Almost midway between the little toe and the edge of
the heel, you will notice a bony prominence. Working upward
there toward the center of the foot, you will many times strike a
tender spot (see plate 21). Work this tender spot out. Then work
down and around this bony protrusion and under the foot in the
same general area (see plate 22).

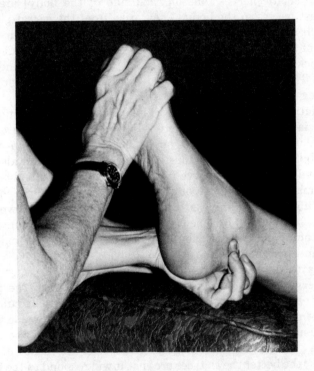

Plate 20. Another reflex for the sciatic nerve

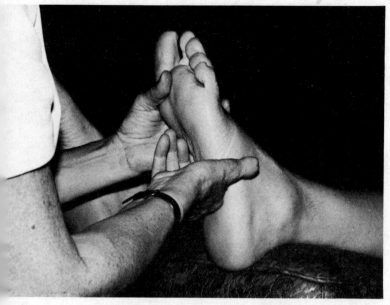

Plate 21. Reflex to hip, low back, and knee

You will also find an area on the pad of the heel, a short distance from the extreme edge of the heel. Work this entire area horizontally, from the inside edge of the foot to the outside edge of the foot, and all the way down to the extreme edge of the heel. If you massage the entire lower area of the heel, you should bring some relief to the sufferer. You will probably have to use more pressure in this area, since sometimes the pad of the heel is quite thick, and you must get in deep to make contact.

In an acute case of sciatica, I massage on the outside the entire length of the leg (up to the hip if necessary). I begin at the anklebone and work up; then I do the same on the inside of the leg (beginning at the inside anklebone). I have found this to be of tremendous help in relieving the pain. I also get into the hip area by having the patient remove any clothing which might hinder my working on the lower back. I take my thumb, place it approximately two inches from the coccyx, or base of

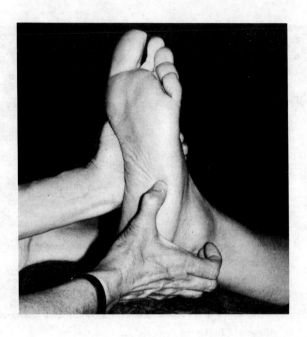

Plate 22. Reflex to hip, low back, and knee
(under surface of foot)

the spine, then spread my hand so that my index finger (and the
other fingers if necessary) will fit neatly into the hip joint, and
press firmly. Deep massage to this area may bring extreme
pain, which can be felt down the entire leg; but when the
tenderness is worked out, the patient gets almost instant relief
(for the position, see plate 23).

One day I took my car in for a checkup. As I walked into the
garage, I noticed the head mechanic bent over in what did not
appear to be a "normal" bending position. I went over to see if I
could be of help, only to find him in severe pain. Immediately I
suggested that I be permitted to give him a foot massage, for I
was sure it would give him relief. Everyone in the place
laughed, for no one had ever heard of massaging the feet to help

68

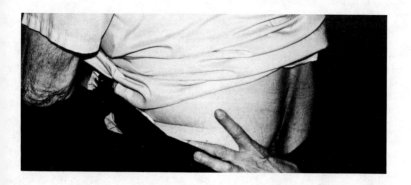

Plate 23. Another place to massage for the sciatic nerve

the back. To prove it would help, I just touched the area behind his outside ankle bone; and as I pressed on it he started to groan. I tried to give him at least temporary relief, then asked if they could get him to my place, where he could be more comfortable. As I started to massage the different areas for the sciatic nerve and the lower back, there was tenderness in every place that I touched. I worked gently at first, until I could get some of the sore spots worked out. Then I was able to get in deeper. When he began to relax I continued to do a complete foot massage, for by then his whole body needed it. After the treatment was finished, he bent over very, very carefully to put on his shoes. I shall never forget the expression on his face as he suddenly realized that he had no limitation of movement. The pain was completely gone, and he felt as though a miracle had happened. I explained to him that Nature works wonders if we but give her a chance. Two years have passed, and this man has not had any more pain or discomfort. Is it not wonderful how Nature can help one so distressed?

# Chapter 15

# The Back

The spinal column is the vertebral column enclosing the spinal cord, which is a column of nervous tissue. It is an important center of reflex action for the trunk and the limbs. That means that the nerves from the spinal cord serve these areas. It is easy to see, then, that a person "uptight" or under great tension could suffer from backaches and even neck pains.

There are very few people today who, at one time or another, do not suffer from that "nagging backache." Often those backaches are caused by muscle spasms, poor posture, inflammation of the muscle, and uterine or prostatic disorders. Also, in certain occupations there is a continuous use of certain muscles or groups of muscles, and this can lead to what is called "professional cramp."

One reflex area to the back is located on the inner side of the foot, reaching from the big toe to a short distance above the heel. The area of the toe takes in the head and cervical (neck) vertebrae, the part above the waistline of the foot serves the upper back, the area of the waistline on the foot serves the middle back, and the area below the waistline on the foot serves the lower back (see figure 7).

The coccyx, formed of four small segments of bone, is at the very end of the spine. It is commonly called the tailbone. Injury to this area can also affect the functioning of various parts of the lower part of the body. It is not uncommon to find that someone is very tender in the reflex area of the coccyx and yet has no complaint. However, upon questioning, you will learn

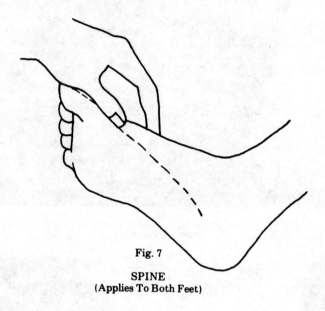

Fig. 7

SPINE
(Applies To Both Feet)

that there was an injury sustained to the coccyx, perhaps in early childhood. This is Nature at work again; for what we have long forgotten Nature long remembers. The reflex area to the coccyx is on the inner side of the foot, a short distance from the heel (see plate 24).

Worth mentioning at this time is a very large muscle in the upper back. Overwork or strain to this muscle can cause great tension in the shoulders and neck as well as the upper back. This muscle is called the trapezius and is the shape of a triangle. It becomes diamond-shaped where the left trapezius muscle and the right trapezius muscle meet. It begins at the occipital bone (the bone in the lower back part of the skull), extends to both shoulders, and then extends down to the nineteenth vertebra

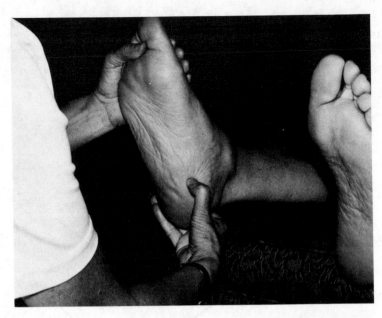

Plate 24. Reflex to coccyx

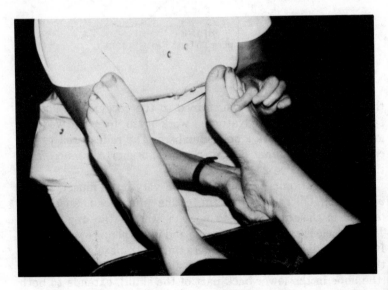

Plate 25. Reflex to the trapezius muscle

72

(or twelfth thoracic vertebra). Because it is such a large muscle, it covers the other muscles of the upper part of the back and neck. If you can visualize this muscle, you can easily see how tension and strain to it can cause great discomfort (see plate 25 for its reflex area on the foot).

# Chapter 16

# The Uterus, Breasts, Fallopian Tubes, and Prostate Gland

The uterus, a muscular organ, is situated in the mid-pelvis between the bladder and the rectum. A full bladder will tilt it backward, and a distended rectum will tilt it forward. It is very important to remember this when massaging its reflex, for any amount of displacement may also interfere with the blood supply to this organ and could cause congestion. If the displacement is temporarily caused by a full bladder or distended rectum, these problems must be corrected in order to relieve the pressure on the uterus. If you find the reflex to the uterus to be tender, then question the person to see if she has recently emptied her bladder or if she is troubled with constipation. Often one of these is causing the tenderness in the reflex area, and once it has been corrected, the tenderness disappears.

Remember, the uterus is a muscular organ, and helping this muscle to relax can often relieve painful or difficult menstruation. One reflex area to the uterus was discussed in chapter 12 (see plate 19). Another reflex area is located on the inside of the foot (both feet) almost midway between the anklebone and the edge of the heel (see figure 8). This area, for some reason, is often tender in women who are approaching menopause or are experiencing it.

The fallopian tubes (also called uterine tubes) extend from the lateral angle of the uterus to ovary. Their reflex area will be found on the top of the foot, extending from the inside anklebone to the outside anklebone. This area also serves as the reflex area to the groin (where there are lymph glands present).

74

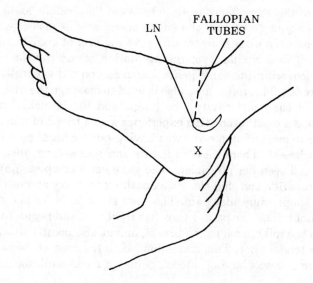

FALLOPIAN
TUBES
LN

X

X - Uterus or Prostate
LN - Lymph Nodes to Groin and Armpit

Fig. 8 Reflexes to uterus (or prostate), fallopian tubes, lymph nodes to groin and armpit.

The breasts, or mammary glands, are supplied with nerves and are intimately connected, by means of the sympathetic nervous system, to the uterus and other organs. Many young girls notice this connection as they become aware of how painful and swollen the breasts become during the menstrual period. Would it not be wise, then, to massage the reflex to the breasts to try to help relieve some of the nerve tension present so many times during the cycle? The swelling in the breasts is just congestion; so massage will also help to reduce the swelling and relieve the pain.

The reflex area to the breasts is located on the top of each foot. It begins at the base of the toes and extends down a few inches. It can be worked either horizontally or vertically. To work vertically, take your fist and place it against the sole of the foot for support; then with your index, middle, and ring fingers of the other hand, work in between the tendons and bones of each zone to be sure the entire breast area is massaged (see figure 9). To work horizontally, take the heel of your hand and work it in a circular, yet rolling motion across the top of the foot, covering the same general area as you did vertically (see figure 10). This reflex area also is used to massage the front portion of the chest cavity, the lungs, and the bronchial tubes.

I had a most interesting experience with a friend of mine. She came to me, telling me she was having quite a bit of pain in her right breast. There were no lumps and no swelling, just pain. She had seen her physician, who gave her a complete physical examination and said there was nothing to worry about, that it was simply muscular pain. This was great news for her, but it did not relieve the pain. I took her right foot and began to massage the reflex area to the breast, and at one point I touched a very tender spot. This corresponded to the area on her breast where she was having intense pain. As I was working out the

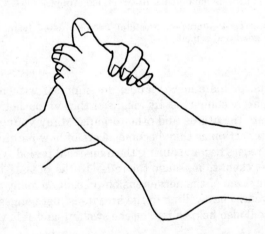

Fig. 9 Reflex to breast, chest cavity, lungs, and bronchial tubes.

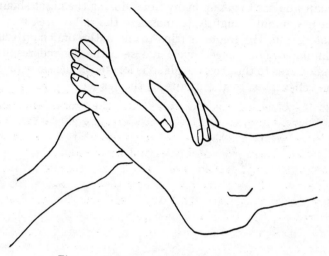

Fig. 10  Rolling motion over breast area.

tenderness, she became so nauseated that I had to proceed with caution so as not to cause any more discomfort than necessary. I felt that she really needed a complete foot massage in order to relax her entire body, for she admitted to being "uptight." I made arrangements to visit her at home to treat her. The night I arrived at her place I was anxious to know how she felt after her "test massage." She was very pleased, because she had had no more discomfort or pain. But something strange had happened to her. After the massage to her breast area, she had developed a rash, strangely enough, on her right breast. This rash lasted three days and then disappeared. She has not had it or the pain since. Since I only did one reflex area on the foot, she had a local reaction, which was confined to that one area. This, again, was Nature's way of ridding the body of some of the toxins in it.

The prostate gland (a male gland) surrounds the neck of the bladder. Frequently, after middle age, this gland becomes enlarged, causing congestion, pain, and frequency of urination;

sometimes, if there is a great amount of congestion and swelling, it will cause retention of urine.

A man who has to get up many times during the night should take a few minutes nightly to massage the reflex area to the prostate gland. His frequent trips to the bathroom could thus be eliminated. Only once have I not seen the desired results. The reflex area to the prostate gland is located in the same place as the reflex area to the uterus in the female.

# Chapter 17

# The Spleen and the Lymphatic System

The spleen, a vascular, bean-shaped lymph gland, is situated beneath the diaphragm, behind and to the left of the stomach. It is the largest of the lymphatic organs. Its functions are (1) the formation of blood cells, (2) the storage of iron, and (3) the removal of bacteria and worn-out blood cells from the circulation. Can you understand, then, the importance of good circulation to this organ so that it may function properly? The reflex area to the spleen is located on the left foot, above the waistline, and in zones four and five (see plate 26).

The lymphatic circulation conveys lymph (a transparent, colorless fluid) from the tissues of the body to the bloodstream. The lymphatic fluid, unlike the blood, flows only in one direction. Along the course of the lymphatic system are small nodes or masses of lymphoid tissue. It is said that no lymph on its way from the lymphatic capillaries ever reaches the bloodstream without passing through at least one node. These nodes act as filters, keeping bacteria and other matter from entering the bloodstream. This means they are a defense against the spread of infection. If there is drainage of bacteria or toxic material into these lymph nodes, swelling may take place in them or in various parts of the body. Frequently the legs become swollen. This may be due to an obstruction in the flow of lymph to the tissues, or the lymph gathering in the tissues faster than it can be carried away by a normal flow. Massage to this reflex area will help restore the flow to normal, and this will result in the reduction of swelling in many areas of the body.

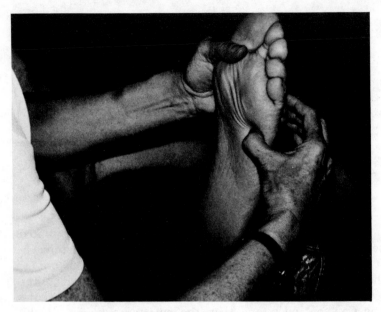

Plate 26. Reflex to spleen

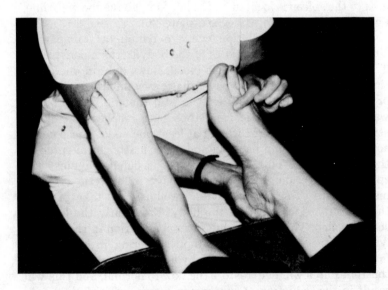

Plate 27. Reflex for general drainage of lymphatic system

80

The reflex areas to the lymph glands in the groin and armpits are located at the top of each foot in front of the anklebone. Massage the area well, from the inside anklebone to the outside anklebone. For general drainage of the lymphatic system, massage the area between the base of the big toe and the second toe (on the top of the foot) (see plate 27).

# Chapter 18

# Other Areas to be Remembered

The eyes are a very important part of the body, and they should be given the best care possible. Although I have never seen a cataract disappear because of foot massages, many of my patients have claimed that there has been a definite improvement in eyesight due to massages. Remember, when you are massaging the reflex area to the eyes, you are improving the circulation to them, and this will frequently result in better vision.

One woman came to me with the complaint of burning feet, and as I did her massage, I found her right eye reflex to be extremely tender. It took three treatments before the tenderness in that area was worked out. After the fourth treatment the tenderness was completely gone, and she remarked how much better she was feeling generally. During the massage she told me she had just been to her eye specialist earlier that morning and that he was surprised to find that the glaucoma in her right eye had practically disappeared. Until then, I was not aware that she had had glaucoma; I only knew that there was tenderness in the right eye reflex.

If you are tired and feel eyestrain, try massaging a few minutes the reflexes to your eyes, and see how relaxed they become (see plate 7).

Problems of the ear are responsible for many uncomfortable symptoms which we encounter today. I have seen dizziness, nausea and vomiting, earaches, and loss of hearing (depending on the cause) helped by reflexology (see plate 8). In the ear there is a tube (the eustachian tube) which extends from the middle ear to the throat. This tube may become blocked due to infection or inflammation and congestion, and loss of hearing may result. Foot massage to its reflex area (see plate 9) will increase the circulation, reduce the inflammation, relieve the congestion, and thus restore the hearing.

One day my neighbor came to me for a foot massage. She was only a child eight years old, but I had given her massages before when she was not feeling well. This day she was listless; and when I started the foot massage, her right ear reflex was extremely tender, and I could feel many tiny deposits, almost like gravel, there. I questioned her to see if she had been having any problems with that ear, and learned that she had been sent home from school the day before with an ear infection. I worked particularly long on that reflex, going back to it frequently during the treatment. She felt much better after the treatment; and the next day when she returned to school, the nurse was surprised to note that the infection was completely gone.

At this time, I would like to mention the reflex area to the shoulder, for I feel that it warrants some discussion; since many people suffer from bursitis or neuritis in this area. I know from personal experience that any problem in the shoulder can be extremely painful and uncomfortable, and the least bit of movement or motion will only aggravate it. I have had patients come to me in severe pain. They had been to see their own physicians and had received cortisone injections, with no relief. Massaging the reflex area to that particular shoulder would bring tears to their eyes. I would work deeply, but gently at first, until some of the deposits began to dissolve; then I could proceed with more firmness. These patients responded wonderfully to foot massage, but some required more treatments than others, depending on the length of time they had been suffering from the problem.

The reflex area to the shoulder is located just below the base of the little toe. Massage the entire surrounding area, including the undersurface of the foot in the general area of the base of the little toe (see plate 28).

Finally, I would like to mention the solar plexus (celiac plexus), which is a network of nerves situated behind the stomach and in front of the diaphragm. Because of this intricate net-

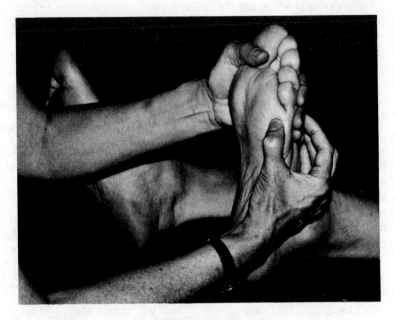

Plate 28. Reflex to shoulder

work, any one organ may receive branches from several nerves. This increases the number of pathways and connections between the organs; so you see how vitally important it is to keep the solar plexus relaxed. If the solar plexus is not relaxed, then you know that the entire body is not relaxed.

The reflex area to this important network of nerves is located in the center of each foot, right below the ball of the foot (see plate 29). The technique for massaging its reflex is somewhat different from the other technique. Place one thumb in the center of each foot. Now push in slowly and firmly, and at the same time have the person take a deep breath and hold it for a few seconds. As he exhales slowly, release your thumbs slowly. It is extremely important that both of you work together simultaneously. You will be able to tell very easily if the person is relaxed. If he is not, as you push your thumbs in, they will feel as though they have struck a brick wall; for they will come to a sudden stop. If he is relaxed, the thumbs will glide in the space very easily.

Try massaging the solar plexus several times during the massage, for this helps relax the body. But as the finale to the massage, do the solar plexus again; then you will be able to tell what kind of results were obtained by the treatment.

Since the solar plexus is in front of the diaphragm, as you massage this reflex area you will automatically be working the diaphragm reflex area. Hiccoughs, which are spasms of the diaphragm, can often be relieved by massaging this area. However, if the hiccoughs are severe, then it would be wise to do a complete foot massage in order to relax the whole body.

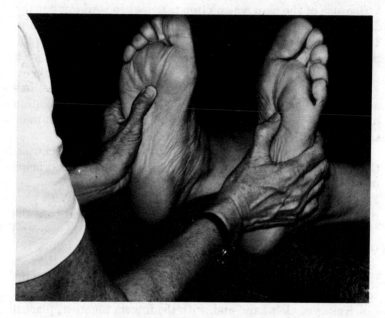

Plate 29. Reflex for solar plexus

# Chapter 19

# Dessert to Ease the Pain

Because of the pain which often is felt when working out the deposits, it is nice to give what we call dessert to ease the pain. This is in the form of extra massage movements throughout the treatment. It keeps the patient a little more relaxed between "ouches."

There are, I am sure, many tricks that every reflexologist has which he or she uses to help relax the patient. I will mention just a few, but as you become more involved in doing foot massages, you will find many others to use.

1. Take each toe, one at a time, and turn it first clockwise, then counterclockwise. This tends to loosen the toes and helps to relieve some of the tension (see figure 11).

2. Take the heel of the right foot in your left hand. With your right hand, grasp the toes of the right foot firmly and turn the foot first in one direction, then in another. Do this several times; then repeat the motion with the left foot (see figure 12).

3. Assume same position as in number two, but push the toes first toward the body, then away from the body, stretching the toes as you do so (see figure 13).

4. Take your left hand and, with the fingers together, place it firmly over the upper surface of the right foot, the little finger even with the tips of the toes. Place your left thumb under the foot, so as to be able to grasp the foot firmly with the hand. Now take your right hand and place the fingers (close together) alongside of the fingers of your left hand (both index fingers close to each other). Place the thumb under the foot, alongside

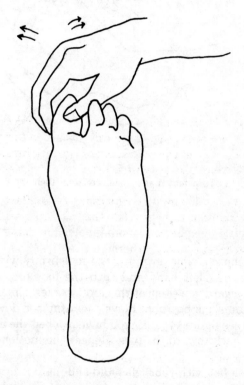

Fig. 11 Turn toe first in one direction then the other.

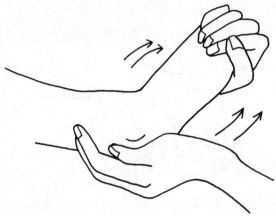

Fig. 12  Turn foot first in one direction, then the other.

of the left thumb. Now, gripping the foot firmly with the right hand, take your left hand and turn the foot first away from you, then toward you. Repeat this motion a few times. With the hands in the same position, move them further down the foot each time (see figure 14) until you have reached the anklebones; then work back toward the toes. Repeat the motion on the left foot.

5. Make a fist with your left hand and place it firmly against the sole of the right foot. Grasp the toes of the right foot with your right hand. Now, as you push against the sole of the foot with your left fist, pull the toes with the right hand. As you pull the toes, stretch them so that they will reach over your left fist. Repeat several times; then do the same with the left foot.

6. Grasp the toes of the right foot, lift the foot, and shake it a few times vigorously to help stimulate the circulation.

Any other "extra desserts" you discover on your own, feel free to use and share with others.

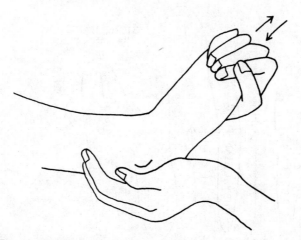

Fig. 13  Push toes toward the body, then away from the body.

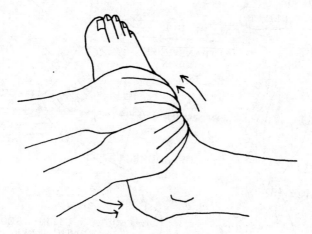

Fig. 14  Working hands down the foot.

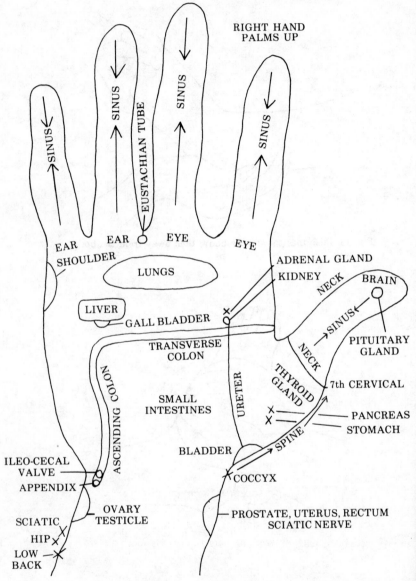

Fig. 15a Reflex areas located on right hand

90

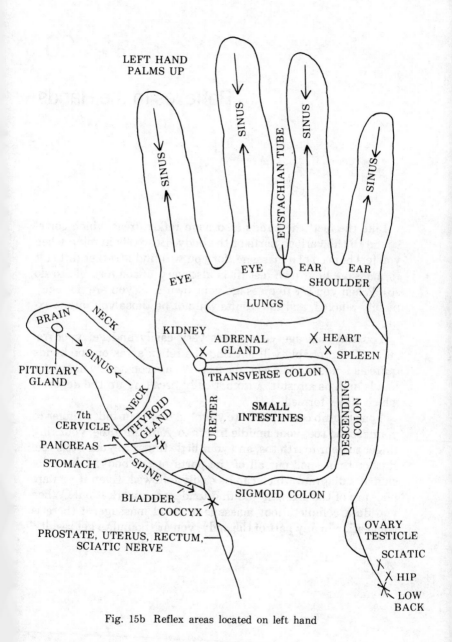

Fig. 15b  Reflex areas located on left hand

91

# Chapter 20

# Reflexes in the Hands

Like the feet, the hands also have reflex areas which correspond to the various parts of the body. Bear this in mind when you feel in need of a massage, for you will find it rather difficult to massage your own feet (it is also very uncomfortable to do so). When you try to massage your own feet, you are not completely relaxed, and the results will not be those you might expect.

You can massage your hands very easily and get good results. You probably will not find the reflex areas on the hands quite as tender as those on the feet. We are constantly using our hands and, as a result, automatically breaking up the deposits which have formed.

Your thumb corresponds to your big toe, your index finger to your second toe, your middle finger to your third toe, your ring finger to your fourth toe, and your little finger to your little toe. Rather than spell out all of the parts of the body, I have included a diagram which can be easily followed. Even if you are not sure of the areas, if you find tenderness, work it out. When you do a complete foot massage or hand massage, if there is congestion in any part of the body, you are bound to get results.

# Chapter 21

# Testimonials

This chapter consists of experiences related by some of my patients. In no way have I influenced them to write these testimonials; they have done so because they believe in reflexology and know its worth. They hope, as do I, that you will at least try this wonderful art of healing. Please give Nature a chance; with all that she has done for your body, you owe it to her!

On a hot morning (3:00 A.M., September 1, 1973) I awoke in extreme pain. It radiated from the center of the lower spine down the back of the right leg. I had to be taken to Pennsylvania Hospital on a stretcher.

The diagnosis was sciatica (pinched nerve), and after two weeks of bed rest and mild exercise, the condition subsided somewhat. I was discharged and told that after a couple of weeks' recuperation at home I should be able to return to work.

October 1, the pain was still with me, sufficiently so that I could not return to work full-time. It was so severe at times that I thought my active days were over. After returning to work in a limited capacity (sick leave exhausted) I was contacted by Maybelle Segal.

She suggested that foot massage might help me, and every three days for weeks I underwent treatment. At first I could hardly bear the pressure of her touch on the affected nerve area, but by degrees the system stopped rebelling against the massage, and bit by bit I left Maybelle Segal markedly improved.

Each treatment gave me greater relief than the one before, and eventually I was able to return to work full-time.

There is no doubt in my mind that foot massage was responsible for my recovery. May I add that at the same time I heard from Mrs. Segal, a viewer many miles away wrote and suggested I look up a reflexologist in my area.

Since this experience, I have had numerous foot massages and will continue to do so on a regular basis. Unlike others who have experienced the same problem, I am able to walk without pain or mechanical help. I need no drugs, such as those they prescribed in the hospital, and the system, with the continual application of compression foot massage, is maintaining the fight to prevent a reoccurrence (which I'm told is not uncommon in cases of sciatica).

There are no words to adequately describe my feeling for this procedure. Unlike anything else that happened to me, it provided the first long-term relief and the first person-to-person contact with the affected area.

Of greatest importance, reflexology makes sense. And Mrs. Segal has made it a living experience that anyone can understand without knowing the complicated language of the profession.

My work demands that I not endorse a product, service, individual or company . . . but I would be less than human if I were to deny the tremendous benefits derived from the procedure of reflexology. . . . I really owe my continued employment to it. . . .

Malcolm Poindexter
Newscaster/Show Host, KYW-TV
Philadelphia, Pa.

Reflex massage restored my circulation and well-being, and many chronic distresses were benefited as tension disappeared.

Mrs. Violet Tanner
Medical Technologist
Philadelphia, Pa.

Reflexology treatments have been most satisfying to me. Tense muscles are relaxed; it is remarkable how many areas of the body respond to this treatment. A feeling of well-being pervades the entire body.

Dr. Allen P. West
Philadelphia, Pa.

I had an injury causing torn ligaments and muscles in the groin, and reflexology improved the circulation to these areas, promoting better healing.

Phyllis L. Otto R.N.
Philadelphia, Pa.

In August 1973, a solid red spot (slightly smaller than a dime) appeared in the inner corner of my right eye—followed with severe pain. I consulted a well-known teaching ophthalmologist.

Diagnosis—broken capillary, no damage, nothing serious. This ailment repeated itself two more times at intervals of two weeks. After that it was constant pain—twenty-four hours a day. I had difficulty performing my job and many sleepless nights. A thorough refraction was performed, with visits to the doctor every two weeks and a change of steroid drops (which raised my ocular pressure from 14 to 18). A smear was performed at Wills Eye Hospital. A staph infection was discovered and promptly treated and cured, but the same pain remained with me constantly. Doctor visits continued every two weeks for nine consecutive months, with no relief. Finally the doctor admitted that he could not find a physical reason for the pain in my eye. I consulted another well-known ophthalmologist. He performed a thorough refraction and could find nothing wrong with my eyes. He told me that I would have to live with the pain. I did not agree.

I was watching a television news broadcast when I saw Mrs. Segal performing a foot massage on Malcolm Poindexter. I had read about compression foot massage and was happy to receive her address from a local health food store.

After three massages the pain decreased by 50 per cent. After six massages the pain was completely gone. I also received a bonus which I didn't expect. I was advised to have surgery to correct a female disorder. Thanks to reflexology this was not necessary.

A great number of people are happier and healthier because of this natural healing method . . . .

Mrs. Theresa M. Booth<br>Philadelphia, Pa.

One day in April of 1974 I awakened one morning and could not put any weight on my left leg. Since I'm not one to pamper myself, I persevered with a limp for days, thinking it would go away. After one week, I did go to a doctor, who diagnosed my ailment as a "pinched nerve in my sacroiliac." After three treatments of cortisone and manipulation, I was no better. Through a friend of mine, I heard about Mrs. Segal and the art of reflexology. After my first treatment with Mrs. Segal, I was able to walk without a limp for the first time in two months. I continued my treatments with her whenever I felt myself limping again. Each time after treatment, I was able to walk normally.

Mrs. Rose Dreeben<br>Maple Shade, N.J.

Reflexology—the shining sun that has offered relief to me! For several years I had severe pain in my legs and back, to the point where it was most difficult to walk any distance. You see, I suffer from arthritis.

Today, after having had the good fortune of meeting and being treated by Maybelle Segal with reflexology, I feel like a newly revitalized person! The treatments are extremely relaxing and most effective.

I highly recommended Maybelle to many friends, who also enjoyed the benefits of her treatments. Hence, I consider myself most fortunate to have been introduced to reflexology via Maybelle Segal.

I have become a strong advocate of such successful manipulation.

Mrs. Gertrude Koch<br>Collingswood, N.J.

For a number of years I suffered a great deal with my feet and was unable to get relief. Then I learned of reflexology and received relief through the treatments by Maybelle Segal. I can testify that I benefited greatly by these treatments and can recommend them to others. The feeling of relaxation after treatments is indeed a good feeling.

Mrs. Anna Oeknigk
Furlong, Pa.

Consistently, over a period of approximately five years prior to last year, I experienced a circulation problem in my feet. The effect was an acute burning sensation, acute to the point that I could not walk a full city block without stopping to ease the pain. The medicine prescribed by my physician had little effect. My understanding is that there are only a few drugs prescribed for this type of malady, and that in a high percentage of cases, they are not effective. Patients in this latter category must "live" with their problem. I was one such patient.

However, on a KYW-TV news broadcast, I witnessed a reflexology demonstration on a friend who was suffering even more than I. A day or so later, I contacted this reporter friend. He was so generous in his praise of the service that I urged him to contact the reflexologist, Maybelle Segal, for an appointment for me.

I have been receiving the service regularly for the past year. The burning sensation has disappeared completely. I am again a very happy walker. Many thanks for reflexology, and to Maybelle Segal.

Gladys L. Thomas
Andalusia, Pa.

Reflexology will always be a mystery to me, yet I cannot deny the results that I have both seen and personally experienced.

When I reflect upon the concept of a correspondence between parts of our feet and our body and the idea of deposits being at points in our feet which correspond to ailing parts of our body, I am overwhelmed; for the whole idea has an aura of mysticism about it.

Three members in our family have experienced relief from reflexology treatments. My twin sister suffers from asthma and has found great relief in her treatments, so much so that when she received a treatment she did not require her normal medication. Her shortness of breath was a nightmare to experience; after a treatment she was able to experience a restful night.

My father-in-law also benefited from treatments. After suffering from a slight stroke he received treatments and experienced after each one a general feeling of well-being. He looked forward to each visit for treatments. Subsequently he suffered a fatal stroke; but while in the hospital, his last few days in a coma, Maybelle Segal, our reflexologist, visited him and gave him treatments. Though he couldn't speak while in the coma, he could nod his head slightly in a yes or no manner when asked a question. When asked if he wanted a foot massage, he indicated yes. This was the last desire he was to communicate to us.

One very obvious benefit that he experienced during his last few days was the greatly eased labor of breathing that followed each treatment.

My own experience with reflexology treatment is equally astonishing. All of my life I have liked my feet rubbed, and never did I experience any discomfort with them. But upon receiving my first treatment, the extreme sensitivities experienced in several areas to my great surprise corresponded exactly to my sinuses, with which I have difficulties; also, the region that corresponded to the low back was very sensitive, indeed painful. This, too, is a problem for which I have been under medical care.

It is wonderfully reassuring to know that there exists a natural method whereby we can obtain relief from various ailments. My experience was heightened by Maybelle Segal's sincere concern and willingness to go the extra mile to provide comfort and relief. With her knowledge of nursing, she brings a unique combination of experience to the field of reflexology that is a source of great satisfaction to many people.

Miriam Niedz
Spring City, Pa.

# Conclusion

I could not bring my book to a close without relating the following story; for because of this gentleman, reflexology is widely known in our country today.

When Malcolm Poindexter derived such great benefits from reflexology, he felt that more people should know about it. Through him, arrangements were made by producer Woody Fraser for me to appear as a guest on the Mike Douglas Show.

I was thrilled and elated, knowing I was to have the privilege of appearing with Mr. Douglas on his show, but I wanted him to have some understanding of the science of reflexology before my guest appearance. Also, I felt the best way for him to learn about it was through firsthand experience. I offered to volunteer my services to the staff of station KYW-TV; so every Thursday I went down to the station, set up an office, and waited for people to respond to my offer. The first Thursday I was there, everyone hesitated, no one wanting to be first; but once the first person came for a treatment and found out how relaxing it was, it was not long before there was a long waiting line. The response was overwhelming! After the first week, I had the privilege of appearing on a local show with Marciarose, which proved very exciting. After the taping of the show, I was asked to go to Mr. Douglas's office to give him a foot massage. Of course, this was his first treatment; and he did not know what to expect. However, he had heard from all of the others how relaxing it was.

As I walked into his office, I found him to be a very warm, gentle, kind, and friendly person. I was hoping that his first foot massage would not cause him too much discomfort. As I started to do the foot massage, I found him to have many tender spots, which would have to be worked out in order to give him the relief he needed. These spots were so tender that he found it difficult to believe that I was not "digging my nails into him." Sonya Selby Wright, assistant to Mr. Douglas, had already had two treatments and knew how great she had felt after each one. She was there by his side trying to convince him that he would feel wonderful and like a "new person" after it was over. At the time, it was hard for him to believe.

During his massage, I found his sinus, throat, and neck reflexes to be extremely tender, and I could tell that he was having pain as I was trying to work out the deposits found in these areas. Halfway through the treatment, he began to relax; for the deposits were being crushed and dissolved and the pain was diminishing. There was such a difference that he felt that I was not using as much pressure as I had been using in the beginning of the treatment. Of course, I was using the same amount of pressure; but the pain having been eased, he could tolerate more.

After his foot massage was completed, I remember the comment he made. He said, "I feel great! I feel like I'm walking on air. I *know* I am going to have a great show today!" Then he asked me if I would go down and treat his co-host, Paul Anka; I did.

Later that day I learned that Mr. Douglas had returned from Florida with a "bug"—sore throat, stiff neck, and blocked sinuses. After the foot massage, all of these symptoms were relieved!

The following week, I had the thrilling experience of being on "The Mike Douglas Show" with him. It was truly a wonderful feeling, and that show reached millions of people—people who were searching for such help as reflexology can give. I received letters from almost all of our states, and also from Canada. In fact, now, a year and a half later, I am still receiving inquiries about reflexology.

That day, March 12, 1974, was the day that reflexology had its real breakthrough in our country. I would like to openly say thank you to Mr. Douglas for the privilege of telling the nation about reflexology—the natural way to better health.

# MELVIN POWERS SELF-IMPROVEMENT LIBRARY

## COOKERY & HERBS

| | |
|---|---|
| _____ CULPEPER'S HERBAL REMEDIES Dr. Nicholas Culpeper | 3.00 |
| _____ FAST GOURMET COOKBOOK Poppy Cannon | 2.50 |
| _____ GINSENG The Myth & The Truth Joseph P. Hou | 3.00 |
| _____ HEALING POWER OF HERBS May Bethel | 4.00 |
| _____ HEALING POWER OF NATURAL FOODS May Bethel | 3.00 |
| _____ HERB HANDBOOK Dawn MacLeod | 3.00 |
| _____ HERBS FOR COOKING AND HEALING Dr. Donald Law | 2.00 |
| _____ HERBS FOR HEALTH—How to Grow & Use Them Louise Evans Doole | 3.00 |
| _____ HOME GARDEN COOKBOOK—Delicious Natural Food Recipes Ken Kraft | 3.00 |
| _____ MEDICAL HERBALIST edited by Dr. J. R. Yemm | 3.00 |
| _____ NATURAL FOOD COOKBOOK Dr. Harry C. Bond | 3.00 |
| _____ NATURE'S MEDICINES Richard Lucas | 3.00 |
| _____ VEGETABLE GARDENING FOR BEGINNERS Hugh Wiberg | 2.00 |
| _____ VEGETABLES FOR TODAY'S GARDENS R. Milton Carleton | 2.00 |
| _____ VEGETARIAN COOKERY Janet Walker | 4.00 |
| _____ VEGETARIAN COOKING MADE EASY & DELECTABLE Veronica Vezza | 3.00 |
| _____ VEGETARIAN DELIGHTS—A Happy Cookbook for Health K. R. Mehta | 2.00 |
| _____ VEGETARIAN GOURMET COOKBOOK Joyce McKinnel | 3.00 |

## HEALTH

| | |
|---|---|
| _____ BEE POLLEN Lynda Lyngheim & Jack Scagnetti | 3.00 |
| _____ DR. LINDNER'S SPECIAL WEIGHT CONTROL METHOD P. G. Lindner, M.D. | 2.00 |
| _____ HELP YOURSELF TO BETTER SIGHT Margaret Darst Corbett | 3.00 |
| _____ HOW TO IMPROVE YOUR VISION Dr. Robert A. Kraskin | 3.00 |
| _____ HOW YOU CAN STOP SMOKING PERMANENTLY Ernest Caldwell | 3.00 |
| _____ MIND OVER PLATTER Peter G. Lindner, M.D. | 3.00 |
| _____ NATURE'S WAY TO NUTRITION & VIBRANT HEALTH Robert J. Scrutton | 3.00 |
| _____ NEW CARBOHYDRATE DIET COUNTER Patti Lopez-Pereira | 2.00 |

## JUST FOR WOMEN

| | |
|---|---|
| _____ COSMOPOLITAN'S GUIDE TO MARVELOUS MEN Fwd. by Helen Gurley Brown | 3.00 |
| _____ COSMOPOLITAN'S HANG-UP HANDBOOK Foreword by Helen Gurley Brown | 4.00 |
| _____ COSMOPOLITAN'S LOVE BOOK—A Guide to Ecstasy in Bed | 5.00 |
| _____ COSMOPOLITAN'S NEW ETIQUETTE GUIDE Fwd. by Helen Gurley Brown | 4.00 |
| _____ I AM A COMPLEAT WOMAN Doris Hagopian & Karen O'Connor Sweeney | 3.00 |
| _____ JUST FOR WOMEN—A Guide to the Female Body Richard E. Sand, M.D. | 5.00 |
| _____ NEW APPROACHES TO SEX IN MARRIAGE John E. Eichenlaub, M.D. | 3.00 |
| _____ SEXUALLY ADEQUATE FEMALE Frank S. Caprio, M.D. | 3.00 |
| _____ SEXUALLY FULFILLED WOMAN Dr. Rachel Copelan | 5.00 |
| _____ YOUR FIRST YEAR OF MARRIAGE Dr. Tom McGinnis | 3.00 |

## MARRIAGE, SEX & PARENTHOOD

| | |
|---|---|
| _____ ABILITY TO LOVE Dr. Allan Fromme | 5.00 |
| _____ ENCYCLOPEDIA OF MODERN SEX & LOVE TECHNIQUES Macandrew | 5.00 |
| _____ GUIDE TO SUCCESSFUL MARRIAGE Drs. Albert Ellis & Robert Harper | 5.00 |
| _____ HOW TO RAISE AN EMOTIONALLY HEALTHY, HAPPY CHILD A. Ellis | 4.00 |
| _____ SEX WITHOUT GUILT Albert Ellis, Ph.D. | 5.00 |
| _____ SEXUALLY ADEQUATE MALE Frank S. Caprio, M.D. | 3.00 |
| _____ SEXUALLY FULFILLED MAN Dr. Rachel Copelan | 5.00 |

## METAPHYSICS & OCCULT

| | |
|---|---|
| _____ BOOK OF TALISMANS, AMULETS & ZODIACAL GEMS William Pavitt | 5.00 |
| _____ CONCENTRATION—A Guide to Mental Mastery Mouni Sadhu | 4.00 |
| _____ CRITIQUES OF GOD Edited by Peter Angeles | 7.00 |
| _____ EXTRA-TERRESTRIAL INTELLIGENCE—The First Encounter | 6.00 |
| _____ FORTUNE TELLING WITH CARDS P. Foli | 3.00 |
| _____ HANDWRITING ANALYSIS MADE EASY John Marley | 4.00 |
| _____ HANDWRITING TELLS Nadya Olyanova | 5.00 |
| _____ HOW TO INTERPRET DREAMS, OMENS & FORTUNE TELLING SIGNS Gettings | 3.00 |
| _____ HOW TO UNDERSTAND YOUR DREAMS Geoffrey A. Dudley | 3.00 |
| _____ ILLUSTRATED YOGA William Zorn | 3.00 |
| _____ IN DAYS OF GREAT PEACE Mouni Sadhu | 3.00 |
| _____ LSD—THE AGE OF MIND Bernard Roseman | 2.00 |
| _____ MAGICIAN—His Training and Work W. E. Butler | 3.00 |

*The books listed above can be obtained from your book dealer or directly from
Melvin Powers. When ordering, please remit 50¢ per book postage & handling.
Send for our free illustrated catalog of self-improvement books.*

**Melvin Powers**
12015 Sherman Road, No. Hollywood, California 91605